HOME REMEDIES

From Amish Country

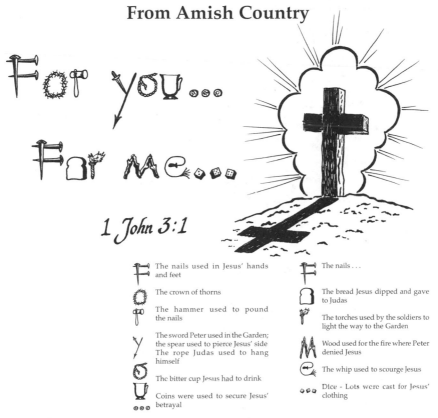

For you...

For me...

1 John 3:1

F	The nails used in Jesus' hands and feet	F	The nails . . .
O	The crown of thorns		The bread Jesus dipped and gave to Judas
U	The hammer used to pound the nails		The torches used by the soldiers to light the way to the Garden
Y	The sword Peter used in the Garden; the spear used to pierce Jesus' side The rope Judas used to hang himself	M	Wood used for the fire where Peter denied Jesus
O	The bitter cup Jesus had to drink		The whip used to scourge Jesus
U	Coins were used to secure Jesus' betrayal		Dice - Lots were cast for Jesus' clothing

ISBN 0-9670704-4-9

6th Edition

Published by:
ABANA BOOKS Ltd
6523 Township Rd 346
Millersburg, OH 44654

TABLE OF CONTENTS

BABY CARE 4

HEALTH CARE 11

WEIGHT LOSS 81

SALVES 86

INDEX 91

Praying that you'll find peace
simply in knowing you are loved . . . by God, and by others.

" . . . my Peace I give unto you . . .
Let not your heart be troubled, neither let it be afraid."

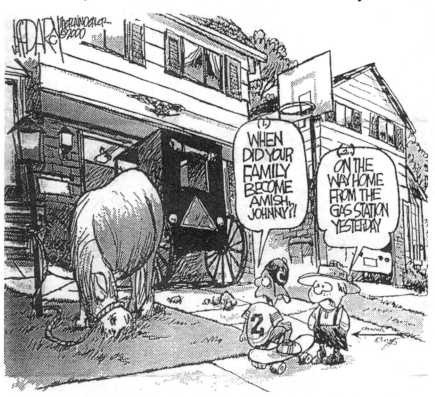

INTRODUCTION

The information in this book has been developed over many years of hard earned experience and has been passed down thru the generations . . . the legacies of a people striving to survive on the land they love. Our Creator provided the "grass and herb" for our benefit and He called it "good". (see Genesis) " . . . the fruit thereof for meat and the leaf thereof for medicine." Ezekiel 47:12. We hope this book will help you enhance a legacy of your own. We thank God for giving us the wisdom to discover the benefits of His creation. We also want to recognize our wives, mothers and grandmothers who provided us with tender loving care and have had a key role in developing and teaching us these homespun remedies.

It is important to note that the remedies do not replace a physician's care or prescribed medication. Rather they are provided as an additional source of information and a possible alternative regarding a number of illnesses and how they were treated before expensive modern medicine became available. We do not hold any of the remedies in this book in harmony with the accepted practices of modern medicine nor do we believe or hope they ever will be. Since these remedies are based on such very simple factors, they are too homely for the more sophisticated spectrum of the medical profession. We excluded remedies that use substances that are harmful to the body or were of a questionable nature.

The paintings included in this book were painted by "The Backroad Artist," Daniel L Miller, an Amish artist from KY and used by permission from the copyright holder. These beautiful full color paintings depict various aspects of Amish life from recreation to the rigors of daily work.

Disclaimer: It is to be understood that the information contained in this book is intended for historical and educational purposes only. Especially children, pregnant women, and nursing mothers should use extra caution when trying any of these remedies without a doctor's advice. The statements in this book have not been evaluated by the FDA and are not provided for use to diagnose, prescribe or treat any disease, illness or injured condition of the body, and the author, publisher, printer or distributors accept no responsibility of such use. Consult with a physician for all issues concerning your health.

BABY CARE

BABY POWDER
For diaper and heat rash, brown some flour in the oven and use it like baby powder.   Ella Stutzman

BABY WIPES
2 cups warm water, 2 tablespoon Baby Baths, 2 tablespoons Baby oil, Mix altogether, pour it over your towels. I cut the towel roll in the middle, put in a frozen yogurt jar. Make a cut in the middle of the lid.   Ammon C Stutzman

BABY COLDS
Put a drop of caster oil in each nostril. This is very healing for babies and can be effective in adults as well.   Mrs. Levi S. Miller

If your child has cold in eyes put a small amount of Triple Antibiotic Ointment (Melaleuca) in outside corner if eye. It will work itself in and clears the eyes up.
Mary Miller

BABY COLIC
For colic relief in babies, mix 2 - 3 drops of vinegar with 1/2 oz. of water before each feeding. This works very well in helping babies digest their meals.
Melvin & Sara Miller

To help with baby's colic, boil a small onion for about 20 minutes in a pint of water. Strain and add some sugar to make it tastier.   Perry J. Miller

For gas, cramping, and colic in babies, give 1 tsp. of fennel tea every 1/2 hour.
Amanda A Miller

Nursing mothers, when eating questionable foods which may result in tummy ache for your baby drink a glass of warm water mixed with 1 tsp. cream of tarter before eating. Low in milk? Try using Shaklee brand Alfalfa tablets.
William Beachy

If a baby cries from bellyache, rub belly with "Unker's Salve". Rub well, and put warm cloth on it . I gives fast relief.   Joe S Schwartz

BABY COMFORT TRAINING
Parental Comments Before Using Comfort Training
"Will the crying ever stop?"   "It makes me feel so helpless."
"We are nervous and exhausted to the brink of collapse."
"It doesn't matter what I do, the crying goes on continuously."
"I don't know if it's congestion or if her stomach really hurts."
"Our baby's in control of our lives and there's nothing we can do about it."
"We did more yelling at each other and at the baby than I thought we ever could, especially in front of our other children."

Over 1 in 5 newborns suffer from colic. It is just as prevalent in breast-fed babies as it is among formula-fed ones. No one knows what causes "colic." Because there is no medical cure, available books can only offer trial and error suggestions.

4

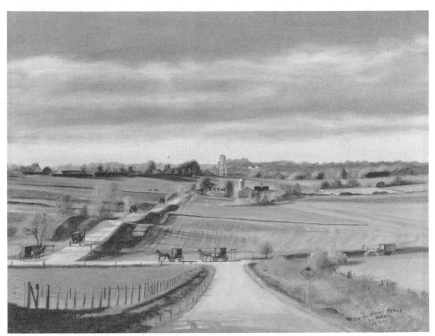

Sunday Morning

X-rays have shown no difference in the amount of gas that colic and non-colic babies have. Did you ever try to comfort a screaming, red-faced and tense colicky baby by taking her on a car ride, putting her in a swing, holding her under a warm shower, placing her on a running clothes dryer, putting warm towels on her stomach, pacing the floor, placing her on mother's tummy or bouncing on a rebounder and finding it lasting only for a few minutes? Colicky babies are trained to be colicky by the popular belief that if baby cries you go to him and pick him up. Colicky babies create a vicious cycle with excessive crying by gulping air and giving themselves more "gas"– home becomes explosive and entire family becomes disrupted. Results: Mothers becoming overanxious, deprived of sleep, high noise and frustration burnout, shorter patience, disoriented– inability to comfort. Character is simply habit long continued. "Woe to that land that is governed by a child." -King Richard III

Parental Comments After Using Comfort Training
"It's like a miracle."   "She's an entirely different baby."
"It's like the difference between night and day."
"We wish we would have known about this 10 years ago."

Basic Needs
Since a baby's normal crying time is 2 hours per day on the average, our goal is to eliminate all excessive crying. You must first satisfy yourself that the basic needs of the baby have been met such as using the following checklist. These are things babies normally cry about and should be met before proceeding with Comfort Training. Baby . . . - is hungry, - is tired, - is thirsty, - is cold (or hot), - needs to be

burped, - has gas, - has a mess, - is sick.

Rules that help babies learn
I. Repetition – give repeated opportunities for him to learn that he can turn on or turn off the music (and other stimulations) by his behavior. Be consistent.
II. Timing is everything! Very important!
III. Reinforcement – we tend to repeat those actions that lead to recognition, attention, fun or good feelings. Ignore this rule at your own risk.
Objective is to decrease excessive crying and increase his alert and calm state.
Time needed is 3-7 days during the daytime only.
Items needed are kitchen timer, portable tape player and a music tape.
Sounds – all sounds and distractions are off: radios, TV, phone conversations, visitors, etc. The only preferable sounds are himself, you and the music.
Stimulations for the baby: talking, touching, letting him see you, music, toys, bright lights, etc.
Areas needed:
1. Sleeping area should not overstimulate him like being close to your bed where he will receive more stimulation by seeing you, you talking to or touching him; he will fuss more to get this.
- Place the baby's bed outside your bedroom
- Position it so he won't see you when you peek in
- Keep the door ajar if you can
- Eliminate any stimulating items such as toys, bright lights, etc.
- Keep diapers and related paraphernalia next to the crib
- Keep a night light in the baby's room
2. Play area is in a different area than from the sleeping area. It is used during the day whenever the baby is awake and alert. A bassinet, playpen or swing is suitable with toys.

Discourage Excessive Crying
When your baby is crying despite all your efforts to soothe him, you must:
1. Turn off the music first.
2. Stop interacting/playing with your baby.
3. Take him to his sleeping area using the least amount of talking, rocking, swaying or other stimulation.
4. Check his basic needs using the list above. Use low energy/stimulation to do so. If he stops crying at this point you may return him to the play area.
5. If the crying continues, lay him down in his crib.
6. Leave the room quietly and leave the door ajar.
7. Allow the baby a time of tension release. Set a timer for 3 minutes. When the timer goes off, look in on him but do not let him see or hear you. Wait for an "opening" in his crying. Focus on the "pauses." Resist the impulse of picking up the baby when crying is for something other than its basic needs. This will be the toughest step.
8. If he is still crying when the timer goes off, repeat step #7. Repeat as long as he is crying.
9. If he has dropped off to sleep, let him sleep. Do not disturb him or turn on the music.

Encourage "Awake but Calm" behavior

10. If he is not crying but is awake, wait 30 seconds! after his crying stops and then turn the music on. If you do not wait at least this long, you will confuse the training. It is not important that you be in the same room. Make sure he can hear the music. Some parents find it useful to use their room intercom to pipe in the music for their baby as well as to check the crying instead of visually checking every time. The music is a reward for calm behavior.

11. As your baby hears the music play, he will learn to identify the signal that announces your arrival. Make your "entrance" slowly and by talking softly as you approach. Make eye contact with him, touch his hands, pat his feet and gradually pick him up while still talking to him. Use lots of happy talk, changing the tone and dynamics of your voice as in singing. Combine these with some physical motion like walking, rocking or swinging the baby. Be loving, demonstrative, affectionate, playful and generally fun to be with. You may want to carry him in your arms or in a front pouch as you move about the house. The music in time becomes the signal that he has just initiated a series of events that will culminate in your presence and special attention. It acts as a bridge between his calm behavior and your presence.

12. As long as he is quiet but awake, keep the music on. It will reinforce and encourage him to remain calm and quiet. A baby can't handle long continuous stimulation. He will let you know by crying when he has had enough stimulation. Parents are encouraged to follow the above steps again to avoid stimulation "overload."

Be consistent and you will be able to train your baby when and how he can "make friends and influence people." This program also works well by going on a long car ride while going thru the steps.

Conclusions from clinical study

1. Music by itself, has no measurable effect on decreasing excessive crying. We know this because when the babies simply listened to a special tape for no reason, their crying remained unaffected.

2. Music affects babies' crying very quickly when they are allowed to call it forth by behaving calmly.

3. A brief rest period following excessive crying seems to help both the babies and their parents by reducing tension.

4. The experience of controlling some aspect of their environment –the sound dimension in this case- by engaging in desirable behavior (being quiet and calm) appears to be highly motivating to colicky babies.

This is a summary only. For complete details and further explanation, background and testimonials for this study visit your nearest bookstore and ask for the book: "Stopping Baby's Colic" by Ted Ayllon ISBN 0-399-515-32-1 Your public library might also have the book on its shelves.

Is your baby a Nighthawk?

Does your baby think night is day and day is night? How you respond to your baby at night will let him know if it's the right time or not. Does his crying at night seem to subside when you . . .

- carry him from the crib to your bed, the bathroom, the living room, the kitchen or a general tour of the house?

- Rock him?, - Talk to him?, - Hold and cuddle him?, - Play with him?

-If you can answer yes to most or all of these, then it is highly likely that your baby has learned to be a Nighthawk. A baby can't change their reversed day-night sleeping pattern on their own. Follow the below guidelines to teach your baby to sleep at night:
- Feed, burp and change your baby in his own room during the night
- Eliminate any and all stimulation. Nighttime should include a quiet, boring, low energy, nothing-to-do, laid-back contact time with your baby. No lights should be on in his room except a night light. Wear a flat facial expression when looking at your baby. Avoid carrying him to another room or touring the house with your baby in search of bottles, diapers, etc. Do not use the music tape at night or any other stimulation like talking or walking around while holding him. If you talk, do so slowly in a whisper; in a "sleepy" fashion. Remember, you do not want to stimulate him during sleep time.
- Encourage napping in the right place by taking your baby to his crib while he is still awake but falling asleep. Make it very clear to your baby that the crib is the place to sleep and make sure he doesn't sleep elsewhere. In time, the crib will trigger "sleepy" behavior.
- Wrap the baby up securely so as to avoid the possibility that his own jerky movements might awaken him. It is comforting for babies to be held securely because it feels similar to what they were used to in the womb. The wrapping in "swaddling clothes" will trigger a "sleepy" behavior. When you put your baby down for a nap during the day, you can discourage long hours of sleep by simply draping his blanket loosely around him.
- Encourage wakefulness during the day by using Comfort Training to stimulate him by having "fun" with you. He will let you know by crying when he wants to quit.

CONSTIPATION
For constipation in babies, give them 1/2 tsp. of olive oil every evening until the bowel begins to move regularly. This may take up to three months.

Mrs John Detweiler

CRADLE CAP
Rub olive oil in the hair every evening before bed. In the morning shampoo it out.

Ben Esh

DIAPER RASH
Rub the area of the rash with Crisco's vegetable shortening. Works very well for dry chapped skin too.

I've found a simple remedy that worked better than salves or other creams. I used plain nonfat yogurt (live culture) and put it right on the affected area, just like you would a salve or cream. People noticed the difference on my baby's face and couldn't believe that was all I used. When I was out of yogurt one time, I tried using plantain leaves. I thought these worked as well as the yogurt.

F Esh

Apply vitamin E ointment or zinc oxide ointment to the affected area.

Anna M Miller

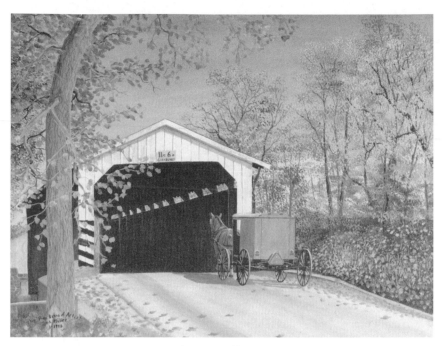

Autumn Breeze

Here is a good remedy for rash in the diaper area that I've used a lot for our babies with good results. Buy some Hydrocortisone 1% cream and Clotrimazole Cream USP 1%. These come in tubes and you should be able to find them in most stores such as Wal-Mart, etc. Mix these creams together and store in a container. It works better than creams from doctors and hospitals.   Mrs Edward Hertzler

For diaper rash or yeast infections, take some white all-purpose flour and brown it in a frying pan. Don't add any shortening to it. Stir it often to get an even brown color over it all. Use this instead of corn starch or baby powder.
                                                                                                Enos R Byler

FUSSY BABIES
Give them thyme tea or catnip. Rue is also very good to help calm babies. The tea shouldn't be too strong. It will also work for nursing mothers to drink the tea. For diarrhea relief in babies, give them slippery elm tea. Honey may be added if desired. Warm water sweetened with honey, given to the fussy baby with a bottle makes them relax and sleep better.   Mrs Levi S Miller

JAUNDICE
For newborn babies that have jaundice or yellow-colored skin, put a few drops of vitamin E oil under their tongue the first sign of discoloration. It helped us right away.   Mrs Joseph H Schwartz

NURSING MOTHERS

Nursing mothers, when eating questionable foods which may result in tummy ache for your baby drink a glass of warm water mixed with 1 tsp. cream of tarter before eating. Low in milk? Try using Shaklee brand Alfalfa tablets.

William Beachy

SKIN RASHES

We always keep Vitamin E oil on hand to use on just about any sore (diaper rashes, chapped hands, etc.). The affected area should be soaked and cleaned thoroughly first and then the Vitamin E oil can be applied.   Emanuel Yoder Family

SORE EYES

If your child has cold in eyes put a small amount of Triple Antibiotic Ointment (Melaleuca) in outside corner if eye. It will work itself in and clears the eyes up.

Mary Miller

STOMACH UPSET

Use slippery elm tea for a baby that cannot keep food in her stomach. Fennel tea is good for a baby that has colic.   Mrs Susie Miller

If a baby cries from bellyache, rub belly with "Unker's Salve". Rub well, and put warm cloth on it . It gives fast relief.   Joe S Schwartz

TEETHING

To mothers of babies that are under 2 years of age, here's relief for those teething blues. Give the baby a bath in 1/2 - 1 cup of vinegar and about 3 - 5 gallon of warm water, plus a tsp. of olive oil a day. Don't do this for more than 3 days in a row. For very high fevers with teething babies, try raw onions on the feet overnight. Onions should not be in contact with the skin.   Ella J Shetler

THRUSH

For thrush in baby's mouth, try mixing 2 parts powdered sugar with 1 part Borax. Put this in the baby's mouth 3 or 4 times a day.   Ella J Shetler

Use this remedy with care. Take a small amount of peppermint oil in some water. Use a Q-tip to apply in mouth.   Perry J Miller

UMBILICAL INFECTIONS

For newborn babies' naval infections, mix flour with honey to make a paste and put it on the navel with a bandage.   Samuel J Bontrager

YEAST INFECTION & THRUSH

For yeast infections in babies or small children, steep some white oak bark (1/2 tsp.) and myrrh gum (1/4 tsp.) in a 1/2 cup of hot water. Let it cool and put it in a dropper bottle. Use a few drops between gums and cheek before and after eating. Also wash off the diaper area with the same formula. You can almost see it disappear. I like to add 1/4 tsp. golden seal as a healing agent.

Mrs Andy Keim

HEALTH CARE

ALLERGIES
For allergies, cleanse your body of all parasites. The excretions of parasites continually feed bacteria causing chronic conditions.

ANEMIA
To help with iron deficiency, (anemia) try taking Vitamin C. It helps the body absorb the food and iron.

If you have a tired and run down feeling or are anemic put 1 T. blackstrap molasses in a cup of hot water and drink. Take this mixture everyday until you feel more energetic.   Mrs Andy J Byler

Ginseng has been used by the Chinese for centuries to ease fatigue. The Asian form, Panax Ginseng, is a superior species. Scientists believe it activates the endocrine glands and stimulates metabolism. Avoid Ginseng if you have diabetes or hypertension and it shouldn't be used with other supplements or drugs that thin the blood.

ANTIOXIDANTS
These days everyone knows that free radicals attack the cells of our body and antioxidants work to repair the damage. While most people know about the antioxidant benefits of Vitamins C and E, far fewer are aware of the incredibly potent super antioxidant power of Xanthones. Xanthones are a family of natural substances that have won high praise from numerous scientists and researchers in recent years. Reams of scientific studies have been conducted on their medicinal potential, since they demonstrate a number of healing properties. Studies show that xanthones have positive effects on all of the body's systems.

Eighteen scientifically proven benefits of xanthones you can feel: anti-fatigue, anti-obesity, anti-depression, anti-anxiety, anti-Alzheimer's, anti-arthritis, anti-gum disease, anti-allergy, anti-skin disease, anti-fever, anti-Parkinson's, anti-diarrhea, anti-nerve pain, anti-dizziness, anti-glaucoma, anti-pain, anti-inflammatory, and anti-ulcer. Fourteen more benefits that you might not feel but they can be measured: anti-oxident, anti-cancer, anti-aging, anti-hypertension, anti-hypoglycemia, anti-immune system depression, anti-blood fat, anti-atherosclerosis, anti-osteoporosis, anti-viral, anti-bacterial, anti-fungal, anti-kidney stones, and anti-cataracts.

What is truly remarkable is that the whole mangosteen fruit, found mostly in the rain forests of Southeast Asia, contains the single greatest supply of these tremendously beneficial xanthones. Mangosteen has a sweet, mild flavor that appeals to everyone. Now there is Xango (Zango) juice, the only product available that carries all the power and benefit of the whole Mangosteen fruit, delivered as a naturally delicious fruit juice. For centuries, millions of native Southeast Asians have highly valued this exceptional "Queen of Fruits" for its healing properties, its premium taste, and heavenly flavor. Difficult to describe and impossible to forget. An ounce of nutrition never tasted so good!

Beware of imitations. Naturally, when a valuable health product such as Xango is put on the market, many others try to follow in the wake of the flagship with a lesser product but claiming the same health benefits. These secondary products just don't carry the punch and effectiveness or produce results like the original juice from Xango LLC will.

To obtain maximum health benefits, drink juice 1/2 hour before meals. Each individual's body has different needs. It may take longer to experience improvements if only small amounts are taken. Some health problems take longer to see results. Your body size may have an effect on the amount of juice you need to take. It is virtually impossible to take too much. Learn what works for you. The juice is safe for nursing mothers and children; they will beg for it.

Another notable antioxidant juice drink is called Noni. The Tahitian Noni brand contains juice from the noni, white grape, and blueberry. See your local health food store or you will be able to find these on the internet also. For a search, type in the key words of the product you wish to find.

ANXIETY
To help your body relax from stress and tension, try Kava Kava. This herb has a long history as a potent herb to induce calm. It can also help you sleep. Do not use with alcohol or prescription drugs.

APPENDICITIS
Use the seeds of alfalfa in a tea to get relief from a painful appendix. Alfalfa seeds can also be taken as a nerve and body builder.   Amanda A Miller

Take a white cloth about 3" square and soak it in turpentine. Put it right on the abdomen around the appendix area. Put a very hot water bottle over the cloth. Make the temperature as hot as you can stand. Let it sit there for about 10 minutes. Take the white cloth off and rub some inflammation salve over the area, then put the hot water bottle back on. Make sure the hot water bottle stays hot enough through the entire process. Continue this procedure until the person gets relief. It could take up to 10 hours.

Untreated alfalfa seed tea is a suggestion to use for appendicitis. Use a T. of the alfalfa seed to one cup of boiling water when the pain becomes noticeable. I like to add some to the mint breakfast tea several mornings in a row. Do this several times a month to prevent appendicitis. Can be used for the whole family. Another suggestion is to take 2 T. of olive oil every 2 or 3 hours. Elevate yourself so that the head is about 12-15 inches lower than the feet. Keep this position for 3-5 minutes. Repeat every 2-3 hours until the pain subsides. Taking flax seed by mouth is very good for appendicitis also. Try sprinkling it on some food at dinner time.

At first symptoms take one tablespoon of Epsom salts internally. Then put 1 tablespoon of Epsom Salts in 1 pt. of water. Make as hot as hands can be borne in it. Wring out cloth and lay over appendix. When it cools wash cloth in clear water and apply again as before. This has been tried and is a sure cure.

ARTERIES
Use 1 tsp. apple cider vinegar and 1 tsp. honey in a mug of hot water after each meal and at bedtime, 4 times a day to open up clogged arteries around the heart.

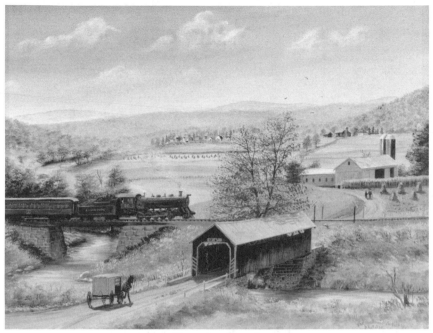

Country Roads

The apple cider vinegar can be taken alone and can work as a diuretic. Apple cider vinegar has many helpful treatments and is most effective if taken at least 3 times a day after meals. Mary Nissley

1 part vinegar   1 part grape juice   5 parts apple juice
Take 2 oz. of this mixture a day. It could be taken for 3 months before you can tell a difference. This is also good for arthritis. Mrs Susie Miller

ARTHRITIS
To relieve arthritis pain or sore joints, take 6 oz. of water and add 1 tsp. (or more) of orange tree or Tang. Stir it well and add 1 tsp. plain gelatin. Stir well again and drink it immediately because the gelatin will set quickly.

Alfalfa tea is good for the relief of arthritis pain. Another remedy for arthritis is to sit in a tub with warm water and 1 1/2 cup vinegar (apple cider) for 15 minutes every night. Make sure you don't miss two nights in a row. Here's one more, soak your feet in hot water for three minutes then in cold water for 1 minute. Do this three times each day, then rub dry with a towel and keep your feet warm.
Jonas K Zook

Raw garlic eases the pain by stimulating the immune system. Several hospitals used this with great success. Chop 2 cloves and leave it set for 5 minutes in 1 cup of warmed olive oil. Fill the toe of a sock with the mixture and rub the poultice over the affected area for several minutes. Sipping a warm broth made from vegetables and garlic can also provide relief.

13

To treat arthritis, drink 6 - 8 oz. of hard cider daily before breakfast. Hard cider is apple cider right before it turns to vinegar.　　　　Mrs Eli L Glick

Take 32 alfalfa tablets each day for 3 months. My feet felt like they were sleeping and were tingly. I used 32 for a time then cut down to half now and can walk well again. What I had read was to take 32 tablets faithfully for 3 months and it would cure crippling arthritis.　　　　Mrs Andy J Byler

Mix 1 teaspoon of comfrey tincture with 4 T. honey then heat the mixture in a double saucepan. Soak a thick cloth with this, apply it to the affected area. If possible leave on overnight. This remedy was developed by a Swiss doctor.

One teaspoon vinegar and 1 teaspoon honey in a glass of water four times a day helps the pain of arthritis.　　　　Atlee E Miller

Mix equal parts of pure apple cider vinegar and pure honey. Take two dessert spoons full of this mixture both morning and evening. You can take this mixture more often if desired.　　　　Mrs Susie Miller

Put two tablespoons Knox gelatin, or plain gelatin, in a glass of orange juice. Do not heat. This tastes gritty, but I couldn't believe the results. Fix this mixture and drink at least once a day until you achieve the desired results.

Someone had a sore knee and took 1 tablespoon of corn starch in 1/2 cup milk once a day for 3 days and her pain was all gone. The corn starch is very healing and will cover all the sores.　　　　Ammon C Stutzman

2 lbs. Epsom salt, 1 dozen lemons cut up, 1 tablespoon cream of tartar. Put in a gallon jug and fill with lukewarm water. Let set a few days, then shake well and take 2 oz. A couple times a day. Take only 1 oz. as this won't give you runs. This not only took care of arthritis, but also cleared up sinus and 10 year old whip lash.　　　　Ammon C Stutzman

ASTHMA

We've used this plum bark tea remedy on our 6-year-old son with good results. To make the tea, take the brushes from a wild plum bark tree and peel off the first and second skin. Steep them in rapidly boiling water and cover for 10-15 minutes. Start sipping. Every now and then, take a pinch that amounts to about 1 tsp. and add to 1 cup of water. You can take up to 1 or 2 cups of this tea a day while having an asthma attack.　　　　Emanuel Yoder Family

Wet a wash cloth or folded paper towel with very cold water. Press this firmly on the patient's forehead. You should see relief in a few minutes.
　　　　Mrs. John Detweiler

Mince 1 garlic clove and add 1 teaspoon honey and 1 teaspoon of honey. This can stop an attack if taken immediately.

A long term cure is to use honey instead of sugar in your diet.

14

ATHLETE'S FOOT
For athlete's foot, apply apple cider vinegar liberally.

Fannie Schrock & Mrs Adin Yutzy

To cure athlete's foot or a fungus, mix equal parts of white vinegar and rubbing alcohol together. Bathe the affected area once or twice a day.

Abie J Stutzman

Put the affected foot or feet into wood ashes for 2 evenings.

Mrs Andy J Byler

Cinnamon is good for fungus. A doctor told us to use plenty of cinnamon on applesauce, oatmeal and etc.   Wilmer E Schrock

BED SORES
Take a 4 oz. bottle of milk of magnesia and add a teaspoon of sugar. Apply this as needed.   Mary S Yoder

To help ease the discomfort of bed sores, mix 1 tsp. of white sugar with a big T. of milk of magnesia or peroxide and apply to the affected area. You can also put white sugar on the sore.   Mary N Schwartz

Make a patty of sugar and peroxide and put it on the bed sore. Put a cloth over the bed sore and fasten it in some way so that the patty stays in place. Another good remedy for bed sores is Saratoga Ointment, which can be bought at some drug stores.

Basic H (from Shaklee) is very good to bathe bed sores with.   Alvin Yoder

BEDWETTING
Try giving the child raisins or 1 teaspoon of raw honey before going to bed. Another remedy is to have the child drink a cup of parsley tea with every meal.

Try adding a small amount of Epsom Salts to the diet. If this is put into capsules they are more pleasant to take.

BLEEDING
To stop the bleeding of wounds, use red pepper. This works on humans as well as animals.   Betty Yoder

This is a great remedy to stop nose bleeding, but can also be used by women who are hemorrhaging. Take about 1 pint of water out of the tap and add 1/2 cup of apple cider vinegar. Soak 2 wash rags in the liquid and wring them out, but not too tightly. Put one on the back of the neck and one on the forehead. Have the patient hold very still. This will stop a nose bleed in minutes.

Mrs Walter (Clara) Troyer

A simple remedy for excessive bleeding due to childbirth and miscarriages is to sip a cup of hot cinnamon tea. Use 1 tsp. ground cinnamon per cup of hot water. This usually slows down the bleeding in a short time and a second cup of tea is seldom necessary.   David W Brenneman

Drink 2 T. of vinegar in about 4 oz. of water to stop your nose from bleeding. This remedy has worked when all others have failed.   Andy H. Miller

Take alfalfa tablets as soon as your nose starts to bleed. Take 6 or more if needed. Another remedy is to stop eating onions. It worked for our girls.
                                                          Lydia Petersheim

Here's a simple home remedy to stop a nose bleed. Take a wad of paper ad put it in the patient's mouth. Chew down on the paper very hard. The motion of the jaw chewing and moving up and down will stop the flow of blood. Or take a piece of cotton and soak it in white vinegar and place it in the nostril.
                                                          Milton & Lizzie J Yoder

Mix about 2 or 3 tsp. apple cider vinegar in a 1/2 cup water. I also give them chewable calcium tablets.   Emma Swartzentruber

To prevent nose bleeds, eat peanuts regularly.   Mrs. Andy J. Byler

To make nose drops take 1 tsp. baking soda and 1 tsp. salt into a pint of warm water. Mix well and administer with a dropper.   Gingerich

For bleeding cuts, put cayenne pepper on it. This will stop the bleeding and take the pain.   Gideon E Gingerich

For blood clots on legs apply warm vinegar on cloth.   Rebecca Miller

Drinking 2 T. full of vinegar in about 4 oz. of water has stopped nose bleeding when all other methods failed.   David J Wickey

Red Pepper in most cases does stop bleeding. We once had a cow which somehow went over a broken off steel fence post. It cut open a vein in her stomach which caused it to bleed profusely. We went for the red pepper container and put it on the cut area a couple times, by the handful, and to our amazement it stopped the bleeding. We now don't want to be without plenty of red pepper.
                                                          Junior Miller

BLOOD POISONING
For blood poisoning, make a poultice of warm cranberry slush. Warm, grated raw beets are also a good poultice.   Atlee E Miller

One day my brother stepped in a rusty nail at his carpenter job, around noon. At evening when he came home, there was a streak of red going up his leg about 6 or 8 inches. Mom was canning pickles at the time, so she quick fixed a pan of hot water, with a good handful of Cream of Tartar in it. Then she finished her last jar of pickles while he soaked his foot. By that time the red streak was completely gone!   William B Kilmer

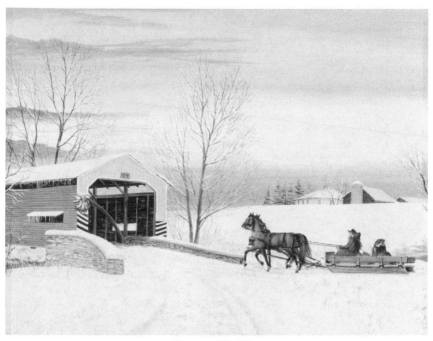

Covered Bridge

BODY CLEANSER I

Cleansing the soul is just as important for good health as cleansing the body. Man has been held in the bondage of misery and suffering with negative, destructive influences from licensed and unlicensed witchcraft.

Cleansing the body is basic for the elimination and correction of every kind of disease. When we become sick of being sick, then we will learn the truth and it will teach us that we can be free from any disease. Deficiencies in the raw materials our bodies assimilate and use for cell building produce deteriorated cells which in turn will produce toxins. Disease, aging and death are the result of accumulated toxins and congestions throughout the entire body. Germs and viruses exist in excess only when we provide a breeding ground in which they can survive and multiply. They are in the body to help break down accumulated toxins and congestions. Do you think that a microscopic microbe which will make you sick when you are well and strong, that you will ever become strong enough thereafter to throw it off? Infection and fever are not caught; they were created to burn off the excess wastes and toxins our bodies have accumulated. When our elimination organs become overwhelmed, our body has the ability to wrap up these toxins and store them away for a later day.

With this understanding, all diseases are varied expressions of the one disease called toxemia. This is briefly defined as a saturation of toxins and congestions in the body. As a person reaches a limit of what the body can tolerate, a good house cleaning is started, and one of nature's most effective methods is to start loosening and eliminating these toxins and congestions with bacterial or viral action. As this

17

action progresses, we become sick and feverish, and the body's other resources kick into action to clean us out as fast as possible. As disease producing toxins are expelled from our bodies, deficiencies must be restored. Thus a cleansing diet must also include the proper material for building healthy cells.

This diet first proved itself in the healing of many stomach ulcers in ten days. It dissolves and eliminates all types of fatty tissue at the rate of about 2 pounds per day. Colds, flu, asthma, hay fever, sinusitis, bronchitis, and allergies vanish with the elimination of the toxins that cause them. Calcium and cholesterol deposits also respond to it. Skin disorders like boils, abscesses, carbuncles and acne disappear. Those addicted to alcohol, tobacco and drugs will receive untold benefits from this diet. Cravings for unnatural stimulants and depressants found in caffeine and cola drinks will lose their appeal. The cleansing has a way of removing the cravings and deficiencies.

Lemons and limes are the richest source of vitamins and minerals of any food known to man. This lemon juice diet has been in use by many thousands of people since 1940 and may be used with complete safety for every known type of sickness. Other reasons to use this diet are for resting the digestive system, losing excess weight, and better assimilation of nutrients from food. Using this diet 3 to 4 times per year will do wonders for your health. Follow the diet for a minimum of 10 days and up to 40 days for extremely serious conditions. All the nutrition needed during the cleansing period is supplied in the diet. This diet does not have any dangerous side effects. Do not substitute any ingredients and make it exactly as shown.
   2 T lemon or lime juice from fresh ones only (about 1/2 lemon)
   2 T pure genuine maple syrup (less if more weight loss is desired)
   1/10 tsp cayenne pepper (may start with a dash and increase amount)
Combine above ingredients and add enough medium hot or cold water to fill a 10 oz glass. Pure sorghum may be used as a lesser substitute when maple syrup isn't available. About 6-12 glasses per day are sufficient. Extra water or mint tea may be taken if desired. When you get hungry just have another glass of lemonade. No other food, vitamins, or supplements should be taken during the full period of the diet. If you do, you may defeat your efforts at cleansing your body.

This next step is very important to help your body eliminate toxins in the fastest way. While on the diet you should have 2-3 bowel movements a day even though no solid foods are taken. Drink a good laxative herb tea in the morning and in the evening. For the brave, dissolve a teaspoon of Celtic sea salt or Epsom salt in a cup of warm water and drink it instead of the laxative herb tea in the morning. This will help open the pores and ducts of your body and accelerate elimination of the toxins. Some people experience a tremendous stirring within. Dizziness, weakness, vomiting and feeling worse than normal may occur for some people. If these things occur for you, take it a little easier than usual. The diet is doing it's work! Most people can go about their usual work without too much discomfort.

Coming off the diet properly is highly important. Drink a glass of orange or grape juice for your first 2-6 meals. For the next few meals eat raw fruit, salad, broth, or vegetable soup slowly. Eat only small portions. If you experience indigestion, take more juices and back off the solid foods until the body is ready for solid foods. To maintain the benefits obtained from the diet longer, avoid food products made with denatured, highly processed ingredients like white sugar, white flour, margarine, commercial salt, feedlot beef, etc. They are major causes of obesity and poor health including diabetes. There is no substitute for eating healthy. (See www.eatwild.com, www.localharvest.com & www.westonaprice.org)

BODY CLEANSER II - GALL STONES/LIVER

This cleansing protocol originated thousands of years ago. The Israelites were known to spread olive oil over their bread like we do butter and were forbidden to eat the fat of animals and were better off because of it. The American grain fed meat animal, fat-rich diet causes all kinds of health problems.

Cleansing the liver & gall bladder of stones dramatically improves digestion, which is the basis of your whole health. You have more energy and an increased sense of well being. Gallstones are originally formed in the liver and some will drop down into the gall bladder. This truth is self-evident. People who have removed their gall bladders by surgery no longer have the painful attacks but they still have problems associated with high cholesterol levels.

One of the jobs of the liver is to produce 1 to 1 1/2 quarts of bile a day. The liver is full of tubes that deliver bile to one large tube. The gall bladder is part of this large tube and acts as a storage reservoir. Eating foods with fats or proteins triggers the gall bladder to empty itself about 20 minutes after a meal into the small intestine where most digestion of food occurs. For many persons including children, these tubes are choked with globs of solidified cholesterol (gallstones, which may actually be soft) which will not show up on X-rays because they haven't calcified (hardened). There are over half a dozen varieties of gallstones which can be black, red, white, green or tan. Because these "stones" block the tubes and constrict the flow of bile, it causes the liver to make less bile which results in indigestive symptoms such as "gas", continuous burping, heartburn, etc. Because the liver is clogged, it cannot produce enough bile to neutralize all the fats in the foods we eat. This accounts for high cholesterol levels in the body which can cause high blood pressure, heart disease, hardening of the arteries, and a whole host of other problems connected to heart disease and poor circulation! Gallstones are porous and will pick up bacteria, cysts, viruses and parasites that pass through the liver. "Nests" of infection are formed, forever supplying the body with fresh bacteria. Stomach infections, mono, back and shoulder pains, bursitis, hives, ulcers or intestinal bloating cannot be permanently cured without removing these gallstones from the liver. You can expect your allergies to disappear, too, more with each cleanse you do.

> Cleansing the body using these 2 cleansing protocols are the 2 most powerful things you can do to improve your health.

You can't clean a liver & gall bladder with living parasites in it. Parasites attach themselves to any kind of tissue and will prevent "stones" from moving. Their excretions supply the body with a continual stream of harmful bacteria which can cause chronic or terminal illness. Visit your local health food store and ask for a product that will kill all parasites. Do this first before attempting to do the cleanse. Periodic parasite removal from the body is essential to maintaining good health; more frequently if you have pets.

The following procedure for the liver cleanse is very safe. In over 500 cases of people of all ages, none went to the hospital. None reported pain. Some reported feeling ill for a day or so afterward but in every one of these cases they failed to kill the parasites first. Choose a day so the minor discomforts of the cleanse won't interfere with your work schedule too much. Take no medicines, vitamins or anything of this nature that you can do without. Never cleanse when you are ill. Eat a NO-FAT (including butter or milk) breakfast and lunch. This allows the bile to build up and develop more pressure which will push out more stones.

Things to prepare:
Buy Melatonin or Ornithine capsules to help you sleep.

Epsom Salts Drink
This will relax and open the tubes and ducts so there is no pain involved in the cleanse.
1 qt. of water   4 T. of Epsom salts
Dissolve and refrigerate. You could add 1 tsp. vitamin C powder to improve the taste.

Olive Oil Drink
1/2 cup light olive oil (extra virgin)   1 large fresh pink grapefruit
Squeeze grapefruit and mix with olive oil. Shake vigorously. Optional ingredients (to help you get it down): A dash of Lemon, ketchup, cinnamon or brown sugar. Mix a few minutes before drinking.

Timing is critical for success. Don't be more than 10 minutes early or late with the following schedule.
Eliminate parasites a week before doing cleanse.
2:00 PM Do not eat or drink anything except water after 2 'o'clock. If you break this rule, you could feel quite ill later.
6:00 PM Drink one serving (3/4 cup) of the Epsom salts drink. You may drink water afterwards to swish down the taste.
8:00 PM Drink another serving (3/4 cup) of the Epsom salts drink. Get ready for bed ahead of time before the next step.
10:00 PM Drink the olive oil mixture you have mixed. Make sure you sleep through the night! Take a few capsules of ornithine or melatonin to ensure that you will sleep! Lie down immediately! The sooner you lie down, the more effective this will be. Lie flat on your back with your head up on a pillow. Lie in this position perfectly still for at least 20 minutes. You may feel some stones start to move along the ducts like marbles. GO TO SLEEP!
Next morning: Upon awakening, drink a serving (3/4 cup) of the Epsom salts drink. Do not drink this before 6:00 AM. If you have indigestion or nausea, wait until it is gone. You may go back to bed.
2 hours later: Take your last serving (3/4 cup) of the Epsom salts drink. You may go back to bed.
2 hours later: You may eat but make it light to begin with such as juice!

What to expect: You will have diarrhea in the morning. A regular bowel movement will sink in the toilet. Gallstones float because of their cholesterol content. Stones may be soft and appear as tiny chaff or as big as cherries. They may be any

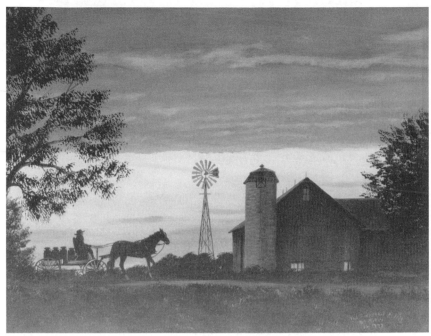

Evening Chores

rough shape and will number close to 2,000 or more in a thorough cleanse. The first cleanse may rid you of a few stones but as these drop down, others in the rear will start to move and drop down too. Do the cleanse as many times as you need to, but not more often than at 2 week intervals. Cleanse your liver at least twice a year. You have taken out your gallstones without surgery!

BODY CLEANSER - COLON AND LIVER
A good colon cleanser is to drink 1 1/2 pints of warm to hot water slowly before eating breakfast. To clean out the liver, eat beets everyday.

Mrs Toby H Yoder

An excellent source of natural extracts, herbs, prepackaged bowel, liver, and kidney detox kits that give you the most bang for your buck is the American Botanical Society - Dr Richard Schultz PO Box 9699 Marina del Rey, CA 90295 www.herbdoc.com 800-437-2362

BRONCHITIS
For bronchitis, take 5000 IU Vitamin A and at least 1000 milligrams of Vitamin C. Once you recover, a daily Vitamin C supplement of at least 500 milligrams may prevent a new case. Another thing that might help you get over bronchitis more quickly is a cayenne pepper supplement. One capsule a day containing between 40,000 and 90,000 heat units should help. Dan A Wengerd

BURNS

Our 4 year old daughter slipped off a stool at the stove and accidentally grabbed the hot saucepan of soup she was stirring, spilling the contents over her body and leg as she fell to the floor. Blisters appeared for the next 5 days or so, some an inch high and 3 inches in diameter. Needless to say, there was a lot of pain and tender skin. Twice daily baths and bandage changes were painful experiences-- hard on a mother's heart. We of course watched it very carefully and were prepared to seek medical help if necessary but because we heard horror stories of how medical professionals treat burns, we were also determined to keep our daughter under our care at home if possible. Through this experience and the advice of our friends, we learned what we would do next time (hopefully never) if it ever happens again. Quick action and proper moves could prevent the severity of the burn and the amount of pain and healing time.

1. Cool it fast. Submerge the burn as quickly as possible under cool water at a sink faucet or in the bathtub. Heat generated by a burn penetrates the flesh deeper and deeper. The longer it is allowed to stay hot, the more damage it will do. Remove any clothes contacting the skin where the burn occurred as quickly as possible.

2. Soak the burn every day (sometimes twice a day) in the bathtub. We tried many different things, none of which we would use again because of its ineffectiveness or the pain it created. The things we had the most success with is using Dreft, which is a bubble bath often used for babies and is very soothing and can be found in most stores. Also add apple cider vinegar, hydrogen peroxide, and Epsom salt to the water. We added approximately 2 T. of each for the first few days. Since the burn area was too tender for us to touch, we kept apple cider vinegar & hydrogen peroxide in spray bottles and Tahitian Noni or Xango juice in a squirt bottle and treated the burn with these after each bath. After a few days, these became too painful for the healing skin. We would instead spray and squirt the bathtub with these in small amounts to disinfect and dilute their strength more in the water.

3. Do not prick the blisters! They will heal on their own. Pricking them will open up an already weak spot in the skin which the body needs as a defense against infection. You may remove any loose dead skin.

4. Use the bottom part of a spoon to apply warmed Comfrey Salve (found in most health food stores). This salve is very healing. Areas where it was applied to and we were able to keep it there with a bandage, healed fast without scars. Large gauze pads with a thin plastic film on one side were kept in place with coarser gauze strips. A piece of saran wrap and gauze strips could also work. Healing speeded up if we let the wounds air dry before applying salve or bandages for at least a few hours after the morning bath. Be very careful to not dress the burn with bandages or allow clothes to contact the burn that would adhere to the old or new skin. Sometimes a long soak in the bathtub is necessary before a bandage or clothes can be removed. Even then it might be very painful.

5. Give the burn victim a few ounces of Tahitian Noni or Xango juice each day and plenty of other healthy antioxidant juices.   DeVon & Mabel Miller

Apple cider vinegar, white vinegar, and vanilla is very good for burns if applied as soon as possible. Put it on the burned area immediately. This will prevent any blistering.   Perry J Miller, Raymond Schwartz & Andy J Byler

22

A good remedy for burns is to make a "dough" by mixing unsalted lard and flour together to make a thick paste. Apply the paste immediately on the burned area and make sure burn is thickly covered with it. Wrap a cloth around it to keep it in place and to keep the grease off clothes. As the lard melts, it will draw the pain and heat out. Change as often as necessary. This gives almost instant relief.

Annie J Peachey, Levi Weaver & Mrs Ruben Schwartz

For burns use pure honey. Apply thick on the wounds, then cover with a clean white cloth. Germs can not live in honey. In our experience this has not left scars if you use plenty of honey.

Elmer Yoder

I burned my foot with boiling pie filling and quickly rinsed off with cold water then kept my foot in pure vinegar for most of a day. I didn't get blisters, but was a little sore for awhile.

Dan S Swartzentruber

Mix honey and comfrey tea powder together as a salve and cover the burn. It will take away the pain immediately and heal in half the time with no scars.

Alvin Mast

If you are working with lye water and your hands start to burn, wash them in vinegar water for instant relief. I also use toothpaste to get relief from a burned area.

Dan S Swartzentruber

Use honey or garlic oil from a gel capsule on burns. It seals out the germs and cools the burn. It will also keep it from blistering and scarring.

Mrs Elmer Yoder

To treat a burn from cooking or ironing, keep an Aloe Vera plant handy. Break off a piece and rub the gel-like juice on the burn. The burn will soon disappear.

Milton & Lizzie J. Yoder

For relief of skin burns, put some Union salve on to relieve the pain and keep it from blistering.

Jonas K Zook

Slice a potato and put some on the burn. The iron and potassium will take the pain away and help heal the wound.

Smear some apple butter onto a scalded area to heal it up really fast. A bad burn will begin to heal and not fester if sprinkled with fine grains of white sugar. Protect the burn from water contamination and dirt.

Henry & Anna Schwartz

Mix equal parts of castor oil and cod liver oil. Soak a cotton ball with this and lay it over the burned area. It's better to use cotton than gauze for this treatment. This should relieve the pain promptly.

Amanda A Miller

CANCER
1 cup blood root   2 cup clover blossoms   1 T. ginger
Pour 1 qt. of water over the above ingredients and boil down to one pint. Strain and add 1 pint of good whiskey. Take 1 tsp. of this 3 times a day.

Amanda A Miller

If you have cancer, try eating parsley or asparagus. These work as cleansers for your body and help fight the cancer.   Lydia Swarey

Take vinegar tablets 3 times a day. When you eat your salads, use pure apple cider vinegar. Garlic is a good source of cure for many diseases, including cancer, if used in time.   Ella J Shetler

Garlic can be a formidable weapon against this disease because it provides powerful phytochemicals which inhibit cancer growth with a 75% success rate in certain hospital studies.

To ease the pains of cancer sores take one egg yolk and add enough salt to thicken as a salve. Apply this twice a day. It will burn. Another remedy is to crush cranberries and put on a heavy cloth. Apply this twice daily.   Mrs. Andy J. Byler

Food can be a key factor in fending off cancer and even conquering the malignancy once it has gotten a hold on the body. Although some edible remedies are exotic and difficult to acquire, others are quite common. One of these remedies, which is available everywhere, is the pineapple. Cancerous tissue is made up mostly of fibrin, which is attacked by a digestive enzyme in pineapple. The fruit should be eaten ripe and raw, before meals. Artichokes are another excellent natural remedy against cancer and are also considered a gourmet food. The curative properties of this delicacy were ascertained by a medical team that worked in Buenos Aires, Argentina in the 1940s studying practical, inexpensive means of treating degenerative diseases. This medical team found that: Cancer viruses were spread around the body by excess cholesterol; and the excess cholesterol in the human body comes not so much from cholesterol-rich food as from a weakened or fatigued, poisoned or diseased liver. In normal circumstances the liver and other glands produce cholesterol only to supplement the cholesterol supply that our diet fails to provide. But when poisoned or otherwise diseased, the liver undergoes the loss of its control power over the production of cholesterol- and the glands run amuck, producing much more of the fatty substance than the body can eliminate.

DETOX: A detoxication of the liver is possible by means of cinearin, an "active ingredient" in thistles. Thistles are consumed by horses instinctively when needed, but rarely by humans because of the very bitter taste. A check of botany manuals showed that artichokes (a cultivated, edible relative of thistle) contain a goodly amount of cinearin. Patients suffering from high blood pressure because of excess cholesterol, when served artichokes, got almost instant relief. The medicos concluded that a diet rich in artichokes might also help cancer patients. (See also Body Cleanse)

CANCER ESSIAC BLEND
The essiac tea blend originally was used by the Ojibway Indians of North America. A Canadian nurse, Rene Caisse (reen-case), learned of it from a patient she was taking care of that had a bout with cancer. Rene obtained the recipe and after running extensive tests, she started giving the tea blend to people she knew who had cancer. Many people started beating a path to her door for her treatment. She rented a 3 story hotel in her hometown for $1 per month and had her patients stay until they recovered. She never charged the approximately 40,000 people

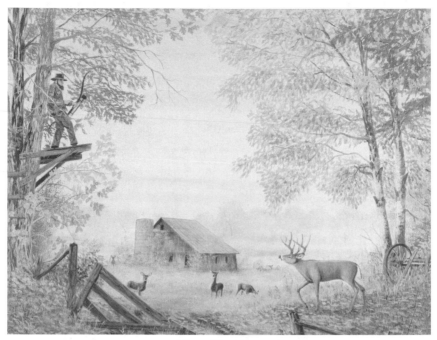

Deer Hunting

she nursed with this blend. They paid with eggs, vegetables, bread, etc. and donations. Most of them were classified as "hopeless cases" and sent home to die by the medical doctors all over North America. The few that died soon after the treatment didn't die from cancer; they died from the damage the cancer or the conventional treatments had done to their organs. Authorities tried to arrest her on three different occasions. (The cancer business is the #2 industry in the US, second only to it's big brother, petroleum.) She claimed the popularity of the treatment and the support of the people was all that kept her out of jail. Before she died in 1978, she contracted her formula to the Resperin Corporation. In 1995, they sold it to the current trademark holder. A few of her very close friends were also given the recipe and formula for brewing the tea.

The essiac blend consists of 4 very common herbs. Sheep Sorrel is the one which will attack and weaken the mutated cancer cells. Burdock Root, Slippery Elm Bark and Indian Rhubarb Root are blood cleansers and immune system boosters with the latter one also as a pain reliever. The herbs are cut and sifted or in powder form. The blend is steeped as a tea. The herbs are potent and can generate different results if not used in proper ratios, even no results. To take this blend as capsules or in any other form is to defeat its potency and effectiveness. It is very important to use the blend of herbs in the exact proportions and harvested at a certain age as Rene recommended, which was based on her 54 years' experience of personally giving this blend to her patients. We did our research to find the product using Rene Caisse' most original recipe and which follow her specifications exactly when preparing the blend. (There are scores of counterfeiters, imitators, copycatters, substituters, fillers and me-too's with lesser products). Log on

25

to the internet and type in the key word "essiac" (or www.essiac.com) and look for a product with her authentic picture and signature on it. There are also some ready-made brewed tea products available.

CANCER HOXSEY FORMULA

1 tsp. Rocky Mountain grape root   2 tsp. buckhorn bark
1/2 tsp. cascara sagrada   2 tsp. red clover
2 tsp. licorice root   1/2 tsp. prickly ash bark
1 tsp. Stillinga root   Mix the powdered herbs in capsules or use in a tea.

CANKER SORES

For canker sores in the mouth, daub the affected area with apple cider vinegar.
Mrs Adin Yutzy

Eat a salad rich in garlic and onions, drinking red raspberry tea afterwards. This is simple, fast and easy.

Put pure cornstarch on the sores.   Amos Miller

Sage pills taken several times a day should get rid of your mouth sores.
William Beachy

For sores on your tongue, wet fingers, dip in alum, and put on the sore. This will numb pain and kill the germ.   Raymond Schwartz

If you have a sore mouth that just will not get better, try rinsing with Epsom salt water. This is also good for cold or canker sores.   Raymond Schwartz

CHICKEN POX

Use Vitamin E oil on chicken pox to keep them from itching so bad. If the pox get too dry, they'll pull or crack which makes them itch even more. Olive oil is also good to use on chicken pox.   Emanuel Yoder Family

CLEAR THINKING

To enable yourself to think more clearly, eat 3 pecan halves daily.
Mrs. Andy J. Byler

CHOLESTEROL

Studies show eating a regular dose of garlic or onions will reduce heart damaging LDL cholesterol while increasing the good HDL cholesterol.

Heard that a doctor once said if you take 3 tablespoons of Apple Cider Vinegar and some A and D Vitamins every day the rest of your life, your veins wouldn't clog up and collect calcium deposits. Also takes cholesterol out of your veins.
Fannie Schrock

Cayenne pepper is very good for circulation and high blood pressure.
Clyde Yoder

COLDS/COUGH/CROUP/PNEUMONIA/SINUS

This seems a rather simple remedy, but we tried it with excellent results. Try washing your hands more often. My children had a lot of colds, even in the summer. Then I heard of someone who washed his hands every time he blew his nose, handled a diaper, went to the bathroom, plus many other germ spreaders, and they hardly got sick that winter. We tried it in our home and I saw a difference too.   F Esh

Does someone in your family have a cold? Soak their hankies in baking soda before washing.

3 T. dry yellow mustard   1 T. flour   1 egg white
Mix the above ingredients into a bowl with a little warm water. Add a few T. melted lard until you reach a paste consistency. Spread this on a muslin cloth and cover the whole chest area. Make sure it doesn't fall off the chest through the night.
                                         Mrs Andy H Miller

This old remedy has been used for a long time with good success.
1 tsp. cinnamon   1 tsp. cloves   1 tsp. nutmeg   1/2 tsp. ginger
1/2 tsp. mustard   Enough lard to make a paste.
Make a poultice and apply to chest or throat. I fold the cloth so it will not fall out as it gets crumbly when left on for awhile. Overnight is usually long enough to knock out the cough.   Junior Miller

Here's a remedy for chest cold relief. Make a poultice of onions by slicing them very thin. You'll need about 3/4 cup. Place them in a skillet with hot pork lard - just enough to moisten the onions. Simmer until the onions are heated through but not brown. Put the onions on a flannel cloth and place this on the patient's chest. Make it has hot as tolerable. This is also a good remedy for pneumonia.
                                         Milton & Lizzie J Yoder

Sprinkle some powdered ginger very generously on a cloth. You can use an old sheet cut to the correct size or even a cloth diaper. Sprinkle ginger the whole length of the cloth, but keep it in the center. Fold both edges in and saturate it thoroughly with melted lard. Wrap the lard-soaked cloth around the chest. You may want to use another dry cloth on top of the soaked one to keep the rest of the clothing from becoming too greasy. Be careful to have the lard warm, but not hot. Go to bed and rest.   Wilbur & Wilma Miller

For preventing and even curing colds, chest congestion and sore throats try this simple recipe. Put 1 cup of boiling water into a quart jar or kettle with a lid. Then, add 1 1/2 tsp. salt, 2 tsp. red pepper and 2 T. honey. The honey is a good addition if this is being taken for coughs and sore throats. Cover the container and let set until cooled. Shake or stir the mixture well several times. Add 1 cup apple cider vinegar. Make sure to always stir or shake well before using. As a preventative measure, take 1 tsp. 2 or 3 times a day. For curing coughs, colds, etc. 1 tsp. can be taken as wished, as often as every hour.   LeRoy Yoder

To help ease the discomfort of a deep chest cold or cough, rub the chest with Vicks or Unkers. Another remedy is to take a large onion and fry it in shortening. Put the fried onions in a flannel bag or sheet and lay it on the chest or the feet. We've used this on our children and it works well. Enos R Byler

For a tight chest or ornery cough, make a plaster of plain quick oatmeal and hot water. I put some oatmeal in a small bowl and add enough hot water to make a paste. Let this stand until the oatmeal is all soaked up or cool enough to spread. Then spread the paste on a man's sock and put it directly on the chest and back. I usually do this in the evening before going to bed and then take it off in the morning, but anytime is all right. This works for both children and adults. This is also a great infection fighter for cuts and bruises. Mrs. Elmer Eash

Slightly cooked onions mixed with camphorated oil or lard, put in a muslin bag and laid on the chest, would break a cold. Atlee E Miller

Use light salt water and put it in the nostrils with a dropper. Adding garlic oil will help cure the infection. This usually works fairly fast. It can be used for infants as well as adults. Mrs. Jacob L. Miller

For sinus headaches, run a lemon through the blender, peelings and all. Eat a teaspoon of this every morning when you get up. Try this for two or three months.

For sinus trouble, put 1/4 tsp. baking soda in a cup of warm water; drink both morning and evening. This also works to help clean out the stomach and settle any upsets. Annie J. Peachey

Mix together the ingredients listed below in a container with a lid. The mix should fill the container only halfway. Shaking and sniffing the mixture often will open the sinuses. Roy & Mae Mast

7 T. Goldenseal Powder 1 tsp. Garlic
7 T. Bayberry Bark, ground very fine 1 tsp. Cayenne

Sinus drainage can be greatly reduced by drinking one teaspoon vinegar mixed in a glass of water. Atlee E Miller

Put a slice of onion on the soles of your feet and wear a pair of socks to bed. (Use two pairs of socks and wear the onions between them. This will prevent potential blistering caused by direct contact of onions to the skin.) Remove the onions in the morning. You can also place the onion slices on your chest for relief from a chest cold. It's smelly but it works. Mrs Jacob L Miller

Give 1 T. of castor oil before or at bedtime. For older children use 3 T.
Jacob Christner

Can elderberries with water and sugar (also a little bit of real lemon for acid). Drink the juice for chest colds or pneumonia. Add a few drops of peppermint oil when opening the jar. This juice builds up the immune system and helps fight infection. You can also buy eldermint from Honey Comb. The purchased stuff has more strength and doesn't take as much as the homemade. Betty Yoder

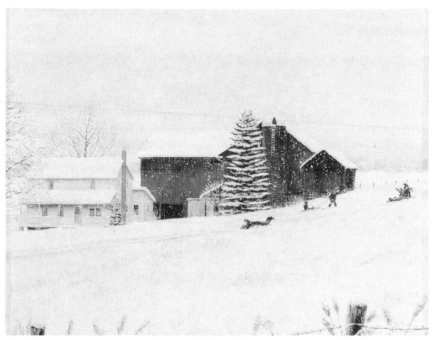

Blizzard

For those nasty cases of chest inflammation try the following:
1/2 cup dry mustard   1/2 cup bread flour
Enough sweet oil to make a paste
Spread this on a flannel cloth, large enough to cover the chest. Cover this flannel with a heavy cloth for the night. When congestion is relieved, remove the plaster. Rub the chest with a salve of Vaseline or sweet oil. Repeat the process if needed.

Taking liberal amounts of Echinacea at the first signs of a cold or sore throat may shorten your misery by a few days.

When you are first starting with a cold, in an 8 oz. glass mix together 1/4 glass of whiskey, 1/4 glass lemon juice, 1/2 tsp. of ginger and 3 tsp. honey. Fill the glass with warm water and drink it.   Mrs. Atlee N Troyer

For eliminating chronic colds, rid your body of all parasites. The excretions of parasites feed colds.

A good remedy for colds is raw onions and garlic. It helps more than medicine.

If you have trouble breathing from a bad cold, put 1/2 tsp. sea salt in a hot cup of water. Using a towel over your head, breathe in the vapors.

For colds, rub Unkers Salve liberally on the bottom of the feet. Wear socks to keep the salve in place.   DeVon & Mabel Miller

For coughs, drink a glass of warm water with a tsp. of vinegar. Honey may be added if so desired.   Emanuel Nisley

Mix 1/4 cup apple cider vinegar, 1/4 cup water, 1/2 tsp. cayenne pepper, 2 T. honey. Take as needed.   Mrs. Susie Miller

For coughs make a mixture of 1/2 tsp. honey, 1/2 tsp. lemon juice, and a pinch of red pepper. Dissolve this slowly in the mouth. Take a sip as often as you need to get relief. The honey soothes the throat, lemon juice cuts phlegm, and red pepper heals irritated membranes. You can also get relief from a cough by taking 1 tsp. of honey and several drops of peppermint oil, mixing them together and taking as needed.   Mrs Eli Bontrager

We've had good results using cod liver oil with some Oil of Herbs mixed in for cough relief instead of the store-bought syrups. You should be able to purchase the Oil of Herbs at health food stores.   Mrs Ben Hershberger

Mix 2 T. honey, 2 T. vinegar, 1/4 tsp. ginger and 1/4 tsp. red pepper together. Add 4 T. of hot water. Take a sip of this as often as needed for cough relief.
                                    Esther Otto

Take 2 onions and add 1 T. of vinegar and 1 T. honey and a little red pepper. Roast this in a moderate oven for about 2 hours and add a little water. This is a great cough syrup.   Dan S Swartzentruber

To get cough relief mix lemon juice and honey, half and half. Another idea is to take 3 tsp. honey and 1 tsp. baking soda. Mix this well and drink.
                                    Mrs Eli L Glick

For relief from that tickling cough, chew on a whole clove. Or keep a garlic in your check and every once in awhile bite on it to squeeze the juice out.
                                    Mrs Atlee N Troyer

Take 1/4 tsp. powdered ginger and add a little sugar. Put this mixture on the tongue, and then swallow with some juice. This will burn your throat, however in most cases, the coughing stops.   Ada Swartzentruber

Put several tsp. of ground ginger into your bath water when you have a cold. This helps open up the head and restores easier breathing. Mrs. Eli Bontrager

To break a cold, chop onions and sprinkle a little sugar on top. Cover and let stand for the night. Take a 1/2 tsp. every half hour.   Mrs Andy J. Byler

For colds and coughs, try rubbing Swedish Bitters over the nose. Do it frequently. It really works. Another cold relief remedy is to dice 1/2 an onion and put it into a pint jar. Add 1 tsp. brown sugar and let it stand for one hour or more. Give 2 or 3 tsp. of this juice to children every hour. For a cough, put an onion poultice on the chest overnight. This will help loosen the tight cough. Another remedy for coughs is to take 3 tsp. honey and 1 tsp. baking soda. Mix well and swallow.

Mix the following and take in the morning on an empty stomach.

1 T. vinegar   1 T. honey
1 T. real lemon juice   1/2 cup very warm water

For cold and flu relief drink this eldermint mixture. Put 2/3 cup vegetable glycerin in a quart jar. Add 1/2 cup peppermint leaves (more or less to suit your taste). Fill the jar with elderberry flowers. Close the jar and shake it everyday for 10 days. Strain the mixture and save the liquid. Take this at the first sign of a cold or flu. You can take up to 1 tsp. 3 - 6 times a day.   Emma Miller

Use a hot lemon tea for relief from colds and flu. Take the juice of a 1/2 lemon and fill the cup with hot water. Sweeten the drink with honey if desired.

Mrs Clarence Miller

We use vinegar, lemon juice, honey and red pepper mixed in even amounts in a bottle. Just use a little red pepper. This is a good remedy. Mrs Joseph H Schwartz

For sore throats take equal parts of vinegar and honey. Gargle with this solution often. For colds, drink hot lemonade; it's good if you sweat. Annie J. Peachey

Take 2 onions, add 1 T. vinegar, 1 T. honey, and a little red pepper. Roast these in a moderate oven about 2 hours. Add a little water. Another remedy is to mix 2 parts honey and 1 part vinegar and dissolve in a little hot water. Add a little capsicum (cayenne pepper). Sip this or take as needed.   Ella J. Shetler

Take 2 cup molasses, 1 tsp. ginger and 1 tsp. baking soda. Stir these ingredients together. Take 1 tsp. whenever the patient coughs. Continue doing this until the cough is gone.   Mrs. John Detweiler

Take one lemon thinly sliced and 1 cup flax seeds and 1 qt. water. Simmer slowly for 4 hours, but don't boil. Strain this while it's hot and add 2 oz. of honey. If less than a pint of liquid is left, add enough water to make a pint. Give 1 T. of this syrup 4 times a day or after each coughing spell.   Mrs. Alvin Yoder

Mix a ratio of 1:1 honey and lemon juice and stir well. Store in the refrigerator. It will separate quickly s shake or stir well before using.

Deborah Moore -Midwife

Mix 1/2 cup lemon juice, 1 cup honey, 1/4-1/2 has. red pepper , 1/4 has. ground clover. Put in pint jar and take as needed.

Make a syrup by mincing 6 garlic cloves and adding 1 cup of honey and 1/4 teaspoon ginger. Let it sit for 2 hours. Take a teaspoonful as needed.

Take 6 large onions and chop them fine. Place them in a skillet and add vinegar and rye meal to make a thick paste. Let simmer 5 - 10 minutes. Put it in a cotton bag large enough to cover the lungs and apply it to the chest area. Make it as hot as the patient can stand.   Mrs. J. A. Hershberger

Make garlic tea by mincing 3 garlic cloves and steeping it in hot just boiled water for 10 minutes. Drink the tea and use the garlic bits in a soup etc.

1/2 cup warm water   1 egg white   A little white sugar

Beat the above ingredients together with a fork and then drink it.

David & Treva Lambright

Take some onions and chop them well. Wrap them in aluminum foil and bake. Give the patient the juice from the baked onions.

Put a wash cloth soaked in cold apple cider vinegar on the chest, then put a dry towel on top of that.

To prevent pneumonia with colds, use olive oil. For children use a teaspoon 4 times a day or more. For adults you can use a tablespoon.   William Miller

Make a tea of the following: elderberry blossoms, peppermint and boneset. This works great for pneumonia, but is also good for the flu and colds.

Esther Otto

Use elderberries for pneumonia.. Take some canned elderberries and make it into a juice. Put it through the strainer to remove any pulp. Add some water and a bit of fructose or sugar to sweeten. Children like the taste of this and are more than willing to drink it. For added strength some peppermint oil can be added to the juice. The elderberries can be made into a tea with the same results. This is also a great remedy for sore throats or coughs, if the peppermint is added. It can help with anything that involves lung congestion.

Take one quart of cider vinegar and heat it well. Find a piece of flannel cloth large enough to cover both lungs, reaching across the chest. Soak this flannel in the hot cider vinegar and lay it on the chest while still hot. I like to use rags and change off as soon as one cools off. Make sure the temperature is hot enough so that the patient can just stand it without scalding the skin. Repeat this procedure until red pimples appear. Works on calves too!   Joe A Byler & Levi Weaver

Here is also a recipe called Pneumonia cure. Mix together 1 pt. Vinegar, 3 T. homemade shaved soap put into Vinegar and 3 T. lard. Soak cloth in it and lay on chest and back as hot as a person can stand it changing every 15 minutes for 2 hours. Wait one hour and repeat. Put warm flannel cloth over wet ones. Wash skin and rub with drawing salve and put on warm cloths. Repeat the next day if necessary.   Fannie Schrock

Raw onions are very good to get rid of colds. We eat them on a slice of bread.

Mary Miller

For a cough when all other fails, try an onion plaster. Fry sliced onions in a little grease until transparent. Wrap them in a piece of plastic in a piece of flannel and put on your chest.   Ammon C Stutzman

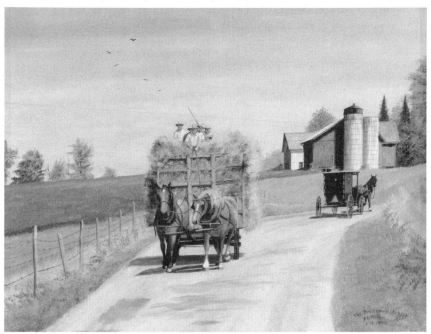

Golden Days

A good remedy for cold is raw onions, it helps more than medicine. I sometimes put them in a bag and put the feet in the bag. Also put them on the back and on the chest. Ammon C Stutzman

We can some elderberries for juice and when having a cold or on the lungs, take this juice and add couple drops of peppermint oil and drink several times a day. Sweetener may be added. This is also good for pneumonia. Elmer Yoder

I like to use vinegar in my rinse water to wash instead of fabric softener, and soda or cream of tartar works well to soak your hankies. If you have a cold they get cleaned better. Dan S Swartzentruber

Fry onions in lard then add a little vinegar. Stir in enough oatmeal to make thick. This is a good cold poultices. Fannie Schrock

Use 6 soft gel garlic capsules and 5 or 6 kelp tablets when starting with sore throat and most times goes away. Can use as often as 3 or 4 times a day or till you get rid of it. Also works and helps when starting with a cold. You won't get it nearly as hard if you keep using them morning and evening for 3 or 4 days, depending on how you feel. For small children, less can be used at a time with good results. Amos Yoder

For colds and flu mix 1/2 tsp. ginger in 1 cup warm water and drink once daily. I had very good results with this. Gideon E Gingerich

This is safe for even toddlers. Cough syrup that is easy. Slice an onion very thin and alternate layers of onion and sugar. Place a bowl or plate on onion to squish it. The juice is very soothing to coughs. Can also eat the onions if you like!

Joe E T Schwartz

Take 1/4 tsp. baking soda in a cup of warm water before going to bed and in morning when you get up. Horseradish is also good for sinus.

Amos Miller

For sinus problems, Boil 1 cup water with 1 T. cayenne pepper, 1 tsp. salt, 1 clove garlic, Cool and strain. Add 1 cup real vinegar. Take every 2 hours or so at first and then decrease.

Simon S Schwartz

Slice onions and chop up really fine. Mix with plenty of honey and let stand overnight. Next morning drain and squeeze out juice. Add real lemon and put in a bottle or jar. Shake well and use as cough syrup or drink as needed.

Jacob Stutzman

A drop of peppermint oil helps quiet coughs when placed at back end of tongue.

William Beachy

For serious coughs make a salve of 1 tsp. cinnamon, 1 tsp. cloves, 1 tsp. allspice, 1 tsp. nutmeg, 1/2 tsp. ginger, 1/2 tsp. dry mustard, Mix with enough lard to mix well spread on thin cloth such as cheese cloth and pat onto chest.

William Beachy

CONSTIPATION
Mix equal parts crushed aloe vera plant and honey. Add a little lemon juice. Take a teaspoon of this mixture in the morning and evening.

COOLING OFF
To cool off and to make you relax in the warm summer days, bathe your feet in cold vinegar water for at least 30 minutes. Use 1 cup vinegar per gallon of water.

Katie Miller

CORAL CALCIUM
The Scientific Secret Of Health And Youth
Scientists report that 157 or more degenerative diseases are caused by calcium deficiency and high acid levels.

• Cancer	• Diabetes	• Arthritis
• Heart Disease	• Osteoporosis	• Eczema
• Alzheimer's	• Fibromyalgia	• Gallstones
• High Cholesteral	• Muscle Cramps	• Kidney Stones
• Gout	• Indigestion	• Headaches
• Chronic Fatigue	• Lupus	• Hatial Hernia
• Hypertension	• . . . and many more!	

Scientists have discovered that the body fluids of healthy people are alkaline (high pH) whereas the body fluids of sick people are acidic. An acidic body is the "bed" of all disease so it could be said that the above diseases are the symptoms of acidosis.

34

Calcium is the king of the bioelements or the common denominator of good health. All the scientific and medical facts support this unified concept of disease, with calcium being the silver bullet for many dreaded diseases such as heart disease and cancer. Calcium makes up to 1.6 percent of the human body weight, making it the most abundant metallic element. As such, it plays a myriad of crucial roles both structurally and biochemically. Only recently have scientists begun to unravel the intricacies that make calcium the king of the bioelements. They found that a drop in the level of calcium in the body is intricately involved in the process of aging as well as a host of degenerative diseases such as osteoporosis, allergy, gallstones, cancer, heart disease and many more. Calcium helps to maintain the body fluid with a pH of 7.0-7.5. In 1970, it was found that the acidic state of saliva was an outstanding manifestation of calcium ion deficiency.

The Authorities Are Talking About Calcium ..
"[Calcium is] A common trigger [that] precipitates biological events as diverse as a contraction of a muscle and the secretion of a hormone. The trigger is a minute flux of calcium ions."

"Knowledge of these intricacies may lead to greater clinical control over intracellular calcium, a possibility that has broad implications for the treatment of disease."

"When calcium and vitamin-D is given in daily doses along with moderate amounts of sodium chloride to patients with osteoporosis, there is a substantial increase in bone mass and a significant reduction in the incidence of further fractures."

"Breathing Easy." "Calcium is required all our lives for bones, teeth, muscle, nerve function, and for blood clotting. Muscle pains, cramps, twitches and even convulsions may suggest calcium deficiency."

"For asthma, calcium should be given daily. Calcium can relax the muscles surrounding the bronchial tubes while altering the permeability of the cell walls, allowing the nutrients to get in."

"Calcium in the Action of Growth Factors", by W H Moolnenaar, L K Defize, and S W Delaat 1986, is an important book about calcium.

"Proliferation of cells in vivo is regulated by polypeptide growth factors. Binding of growth factors to their specific cell-surface receptors initiates a cascade of biochemical events in the cell, which ultimately leads to deoxyribonucleic acid (DNA) synthesis and cell division. The immediate consequence of receptor activation includes a sustained increase in cytoplasm pH and a transient rise in cytoplasm-free calcium ions. These suggest that the rise in calcium ions is indispensable for cell proliferation."

"How a Mineral Can Vitalize Your Health", by Dr. James K. Van Fleet, in the book Magic of Catalytic Health Vitalizers 1980, Parker Publishing, is an important book about calcium.

Dr. Henry C. Sherman, the noted biochemist, has stated in effect that the prime period of human life could be extended by a moderate increase in calcium in the diet.

"When the body does not get enough calcium, it will withdraw what little calcium it has from the bones to make sure there is enough in the blood stream."

"The connection between the electrical activity of the cell and the release of the neurotransmitter is not direct; an essential intermediary is the calcium ion."

"Calcium has been recognized as a major regulatory ion in all living organisms."

"Considering the wide variety of calcium binding proteins in the cell the potential targets of calcium-related disorders are enormous."

"The regulation of mitosis and cell division is one of the fundamental questions of cell biology. Calcium has been implicated as a regulatory factor in both."

"World-class scientists are concluding that there is a link between calcium deficiency and cancer. Calcium deficiency in the body fluids outside and inside of the cell stimulates the proliferation of both virus and cell mutation-- cancer, by regulating DNA synthesis."

"Calcium must certainly be the major bioelement of the times. Today we know dozens, if not hundreds, of different cellular and extracellular processes that are regulated by the changes in cytosolic or extracellular calcium, ions.

"As we have seen, calcium is central to the ordered progression of replicating cells through their growth-division cycle. Calcium is specifically required for spreading. Lowering the extracellular calcium and preventing spreading both block the initiation of DNA synthesis, without stopping ongoing DNA synthesis. Calcium may be the key to understand cancer."

"A number of important metabolic processes are influenced by small changes in extracellular ionized calcium concentration. These include: (a) the excitability of nerve function and neural transmission; (b) the secretion by cells of proteins and hormones, etc., (c) the coupling of cell excitation with cell response; (d) cell proliferation; (e) blood coagulation; (f) maintenance of the stability and permeability of cell members; (g) modulation of activity, in particular those enzymes involved in glycogenolysis; and (h) the mineralization of newly formed bone."

"The early work of Otto Wartburg (Nobel Prize Winner), some 60 years ago, showed clearly that cancer was associated with anaerobic (deficiency of oxygen) conditions, resulting in fermentation and a drop in the pH level of the cell. Moreover the production of mutation receptors cannot occur with the pH of the cell in the healthy, calcium buffered 7.4 - 6.6 range."

"At the beginning of the Twentieth Century, calcium was known by biologists and physiologists to be a component of bone material, and little else. Then it was

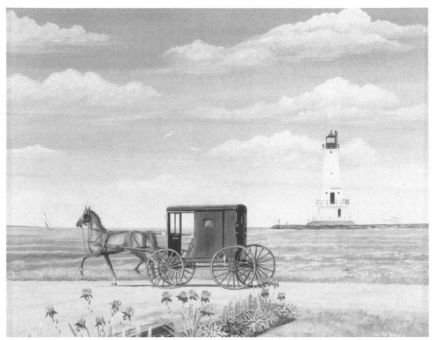

Lighthouse

discovered as a necessary constituent of blood plasma required in blood coagulation and heart function. Only a few, such as Baird Hastings, Walter Heibrunn and Carl Reich, saw more clearly into the future of the calcium ion as a total body health factor, a future that would be a long time coming. From the beginning of Dr. Reich's medical practice, he began by immediately recognizing that many of the medical ailments of which his patients were complaining, were accompanied by what he suspected was deficiency in ionized calcium.

The first significant work about calcium was done in the late 1950's and early 1960's by A.L. Hodgkin and A.F. Huxley, for which they won Nobel Prize in 1963. They researched and measured the means by which the nerve cell membrane is electrically charged and discharged. Calcium ion was later shown by other researchers to play an integral role in this process. In the 1970's, the scientific world witnessed a crescendo of biological calcium research. In 1982, Rodolfo R. Linas, while researching calcium is synoptic transmission was able to explain how a current of calcium ions triggers the passage of signals from one nerve cell to another, the process of electrical nerve stimuli. By 1985, Carafoli and Penniston had further studied the importance of the calcium ion in controlling biochemical processes. By 1986, Moolenaor, Defize and Delaat had found that the rise in calcium ions is indispensable for cell proliferation. By 1988, Marvin P. Thompson is summarizing that calcium is a major regulatory ion in all-living organisms, interest in calcium is in the logarithmic phase, and calcium related disorders are enormous. By 1990, thousands of publications and books had been written extolling the importance of the calcium factors in the human body.

Additional information about the calcium factor may be obtained in the following: The Chemistry of Calcium, Calcium and Digestion, The Calcium Cycle, Calcium and Cancer, Dr. Reich Concept of Diseases and Calcium, and Calcium and Electromagnetism.

World's Oldest Living Man Is Documented By the Guinness Book of World Records

Several centuries ago coral calcium from Okinawa was sold in the first drugstore that was established in the world. Said drugstore is a museum at the present time and is located in Madrid, Spain. Ship captains would travel to Okinawa, load their ship with Coral Calcium, take it home and sell it for more than its weight in gold.

In 1979, a British journalist from Guinness Book of World Records went on assignment to the islands of Okinawa off the coast of Japan to interview Shigechiyo Izumi, the world's oldest documented living person. What he found was a man 115 years old with remarkably good health and vitality who had worked regularly until the age of 105. Investigating further, the journalist discovered Mr. Izumi was not the exception. Most of the island's inhabitants were physically fit, had low incidences of serious illness and enjoyed long lifespans. The population is close to 4.5 million and 38% of them reach the age of 100. Interested in studying this further, the journalist persuaded Mr. Izumi to submit to a medical check-up. The results were even more amazing. How could a person of his age possibly be so healthy?

Soon, a team of researchers arrived and made an important discovery. They found that all the islanders had one thing in common. The water they drank was different from water found anywhere else in the world! The key was to find why the water was so different. They learned these particular islands were built up from the coral reefs like so many other islands. But there was a difference. These coral reefs weren't found anywhere else in the world. The reefs were Sango Coral, the only coral out of 2,500 species with life-giving benefits. A study of Sango Coral shows it is composed of calcium, magnesium, sodium, potassium and many other essential trace minerals and microscopic elements essential to human life. The composition of the Sango Coral is identical to that of the human skeleton and is widely used for bone grafts throughout the world.

Robert Barefoot explains in one of his seminars how the team of researchers were led to discover the key to good health from Coral Calcium. The researchers saw chickens pecking the coral rocks. They laid twice as many eggs than chickens normally do and they were delicious. The dairy cows which licked the Sango Coral reefs gave twice as much milk than others did and their milk was delicious.

Coral Calcium Turns Water Alkaline For Healthy pH Balance In The Body

It was learned that by adding a small amount of this Coral Calcium to ordinary drinking water an alkaline pH of 7.5 to 8.5 is achieved. Scientists have long known that the maintenance of an alkaline pH is critical to cellular health. Optimum alkalinity of the cellular level equates to optimum health. The "King of Minerals", is immediately bioavailable to the body in ionic form. The calcium and minerals in Coral Calcium become ionic in the water and are promptly 100% bioavailable

to the cells. This was a major discovery due to the importance of calcium in the body. It is scientifically documented that up to 157 diseases are related to calcium deficiency. For this reason, it is often called the "King of Minerals". But in order for calcium to do its work, the body must convert it to an ionic form (1,000 times smaller than collodial) or the calcium is not utilized. That problem is solved as the calcium becomes ionic immediately for use by the body. Use of Coral Calcium obtained from Sango Coral will assist in the following: (a) Assimilate vitamins and minerals from the food you eat and the supplement you take; (b) Combat arthritis, heart disease and other illnesses; (c) Absorb and use available calcium; (d) Cleanse the kidneys, intestines and liver by breaking down heavy metals, toxins and drug residues in your body; (e) Protect your body from free radical damage; (f) Increase muscle and joint mobility; (g) Increase your oxygen levels; (h) Control digestive problems; (i) Regulate blood sugar; j) Manage blood pressure; (k) Neutralize harmful acids that leads to illness.
By: Raul Feliciano Arieta, MD License #1857 January 8, 2000.

About Coral Calcium Plus - Secrets from the ocean, the secret of longevity
Calcium levels impact many functions of the body, including organ function, skeletal strength, and resisting disease. Proper alkaline pH balance helps the body better utilize other minerals and vitamins, which is with unpredictable diets. Easier to take then bulky calcium supplements.

Not all coral cacium is born equal. Coral Calcium Plus comes from Sango Coral, and is more bioavailable than any other form of calcium. Calcium helps perfect the alkaline pH balance of the body, and the water we drink. Among the oldest and most primitive of organisms is coral. Coral reefs surround islands everywhere in the world, but the coral reefs surrounding Okinawa have proved to be like no other. Out of over 2,500 varieties of coral in the world, only the Sango Coral contains a perfectly balanced ratios of organic composition identical to that of the human skeleton, including calcium, magnesium, sodium, potassium as well as almost 70 other trace minerals essential to human life. After years of research, scientists found that just a small amount of these special coral sands, when added to just about any liquid, bring it to an alkaline pH balance of 7.5 to 8.5, which is necessary for facilitating optimum health and the absorption of vitamins and minerals. Because the gradual acidity of the water we drink contributes to the development of degenerative disease, this was an important discovery.

Coral Calcium Plus, taken with water, becomes ionic, and therefore becomes (100%) immediately bioavailable to the body's cells, unlike typical calcium supplements (5% bioavailble and 20% bioavailable for chelated supplements). Taken three times a day with water, Coral Calcium Plus delivers critical calcium—otherwise tough to absorb and be used effectively by the body—and over 60 critical minerals to your system. Often called "the king of the minerals," calcium is considered the common denominator of good health. While calcium has been noted for its value in preserving the structure of the body, recent research links appropriate calcium levels to the process of aging as well as many degenerative diseases such as osteoporosis, allergies, gallstone disease, heart disease, cancer and many more.

Results From CORAL CALCIUM
"I was diagnosed with Chronic Fatigue Syndrome and chronic allergies 25 years

ago. I've been told I have the Epstein Bar virus. When I started on the Coral Calcium, I was very tired, but from day one, I picked up energy. Now I can go all day long -just go. I do not feel tired. I am very happy about it. -Ruth B., DE

"After a serious accident a few years ago, I developed arthritis and fybromyalgia. After just a few weeks on the Coral Calcium, 95% of the pain was gone and my mobility was restored. I not only have my life back but my daughter has her mother back!" - Connie K., MI

"I was diagnosed with Multiple Sclerosis in 1978, and along with the disease came excruciating pain. In 1986, a pump was surgically installed in my abdomen, which put morphine into my spinal fluid 24 hours a day. Last year, after nine times in the hospital and eight surgeries, someone introduced me to colloidal minerals which began to turn my life around, but did not alleviate the pain. When I heard about the Coral Calcium, I thought, "How is a calcium product going to help me?" Well, I first tried it on June 24th and it didn't take me long to realize that this was not the run-of-the-mill calcium! About the first of July I realized that I had no pain! For the first time in 19 years I can work 12 hours a day without stopping to lie down."   -Dr. Bailey, OH

"For over 20 years I have experienced severe leg cramps. The doctor told me what I needed was more calcium. I tried calcium of every kind - prescription, over-the-counter, even natural calcium. A doctor even began giving me intravenous calcium because the cramps were so bad, but it never completely eliminated the pain. The problem got so bad that my sleep was disturbed terribly. After just a few days of drinking the Coral Calcium water, my leg cramps were gone. Talk about relief!"   -Cecelia B., AZ

"Three years ago, I fell on some ice and I broke my ankle. I am a nurse, and last year in September after a very hard shift, I was diagnosed by a doctor as having arthritis. My ankle swelled up so much that I just couldn't get around. When you work in a very busy hospital, you've got to keep going. I was so surprised when in July I started on the Coral Calcium. I am now able to keep up with everybody else and I walk a good five to ten miles a day! In September of this year, I had a doctor re-examine my leg --he was amazed to find out that I no longer have arthritis in my ankle!"   -Gail 0., WI

For more stories on how Coral Calcium has benefitted others, see **www.cureamerica.net.**

Farming With Calcium
Good farmers and gardeners know it is important to add Hi-Calcium lime to the soil so field crops and garden produce are able to absorb the proper amount of nutrients from the soil. If the pH in the soil is at the proper level their crops and produce will do well and pest problems will be minimized. Hi-Calcium lime is used to accomplish this. Good farmers also know that to keep their cattle healthy, they need proper nutrients in their diet. Cattle need feed raised on properly balanced soil and a supply of bioavailable calcium or they become chronically sick, have constant problems with parasites and become an economic liability to the farmer. Doesn't it make sense that the same would be true for us?

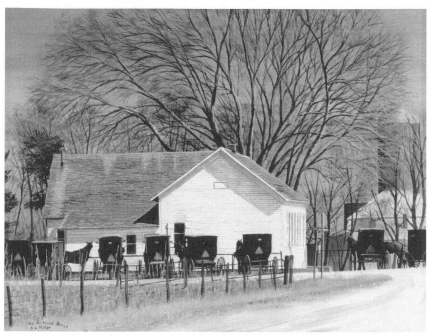

Meeting

Calcium Deficiency and Disease

An estimated 60.8 million American Americans have one or more forms of cardiovascular disease. -American Heart Association, 2001

According to the Arthritus Foundation, osteoarthritus is the most common form of arthritus, afflicting an estimated 20.7 million Americans. -USA Today, September 13, 2001

25-30 million Americans are diagnosed with low bone mineral density. -Consensus Developement Conf. Am J Med 94:646. 1993

25% of senior women who suffer a hip fracture die within one year from complications. -Women's Health 6;661 1997

Disease and pain can flourish in an acidic environment. As water douses fire, so calcium will douse the acid in our bodies. Eating food grown in mineral depleted soils contributes to the increased rate of disease today. In 1900, 3% of Americans had an incidence of cancer. In 2000, the rate is 38%. At this pace, by the end of the next century, 100% of Americans will get cancer. Diabetes has risen 400% in the last 20 years. Alzheimer's now strikes 50% of the people over age 70. Sixty years ago it didn't exist. Most degenerative diseases develope within a window of 5 years. Are you developing one of these? According to Robert Barefoot, scientist and expert on the effects of calcium on the human body, you could get enough calcium each day if you ate . . . 2 gallons of milk AND 23 lbs. of spinach AND 17 lbs. of broccoli AND 23 lbs. of cabbage OR take a good bioavailable Coral Calcium.

More Bang For Your Buck!
Most other calciums on the market are only 7%-21% absorbable or bioavailable to your body with synthetic components added. The actual amount of calcium contained in a bottle useable by your body is very small. Coral Calcium is 90%-100% bioavailable. Even though Coral Calcium is rather new in the USA, many users love the dramatic health benefits they are already experiencing. Some will experience relief of symptoms in just a few days, especially the young. For the middle aged, it may take four months or longer depending on each individual's health condition. For the elderly it could take a year or more to shake all the accumulated toxins loose; again this depends on the individual's health condition. The journey to good health starts with the first step in correcting the problem. Remember, calcium is the most abundant mineral in our body. It is responsible for many of the functions of our teeth, muscle movement, heartbeat, etc. These are all dependent on a sufficient calcium and mineral supply.

Whose Coral Calcium Should I Use?
With all the different Coral Calcium brands today, how can you know which is the pure and authentic one? There are scores of counterfeits, imitations, copycats, substitutes to which fillers and synthetic elements are added to produce a cheaper product. The products from these companies may render themselves ineffective and do nothing for your health. A scientist confirmed the most pristine, natural and effective coral calcium is mined "above ocean" and the calcium to magnesium ratio is 2:1 in its natural state. The Coral Calcium from Vision For Life meets both of these criteria plus it has over 70 trace minerals which occur in their natural form.

TAKE CHARGE OF YOUR OWN HEALTH TODAY!
Take charge of your own health like thousands of others have already done. Some people see huge results in 2-3 days. For others it takes 2-3 months before they see any dramatic results. Take the recommended dosage or find what amount works best for you. Some elderly people in poor health take up to 9 per day. Others in fair health take only 1 or 2 per day. Unlike many other supplements, you won't need to wonder if Coral Calcium is doing something for you or not. Let's not kid ourselves, though. Our bodies have the ability to "wrap up" toxins, drug residues, and other foreign matter in our cells. After a lifetime of accumulating these, we aren't going to be in excellent health overnight. You might even become "sick" with a health crisis because of all the toxins that the calcium will shake loose and your body can't eliminate fast enough. Rest assured that the calcium is doing it's work. If this happens, ease off the amount of calcium you take for awhile so your body can handle the rate of elimination. After a time you may slowly increase your intake again. Happy living!

These statements have not been evaluated by the FDA and are not provided for use to diagnose, prescribe or treat any disease, illness or injured condition of the body.

Coral Calcium - Each bottle contains 90 capsules; recommended dosage is 1 with each meal; 3 capsules contain 801 mg of Calcium balanced with proper amounts of Magnesium and other nutrients. Suggested Retail $36. For ordering a supply at a reduced price send check or money order of $26 per bottle plus $2 shipping & handling, 75¢ each additional to:
Mose Miller 5690A County Rd 333 Millersburg, OH 44654 330-464-2555

DEPRESSION
St John's Wort is effective in chasing away your mild to moderate gloomies.

DIARRHEA
Dehydration is something to be very cautious of in both children and adults.
Pedialyte to prevent dehydration

1/4 tsp. Soda	1/4 tsp. Salt	1 T. Sugar

Boil 1 qt. of water flavor with jello. Give for nausea. They will not throw up if they drink this. Let them drink all they can and want. This recipe comes from a nurse who used it for her children and it really does work. Junior Miller & David J Wickey & Simon S Schwartz & Joe S Schwartz

To cure diarrhea, drink 1 cup of blackberry or blueberry juice, twice a day.
Mrs. Andy J. Byler

For treatment of diarrhea, bring milk to the boiling point and then let cool a little. Pour the still warm milk over soda crackers and eat.
Mrs. Glen H. Lambright

Canned blackberry juice is very good for diarrhea. Can the blackberries as you normally would, then drink the juice.   Mrs Elmer Yoder

Gather strawberry leaves and make a tea. Drink some of this every so often until the diarrhea is better.   Anna M Miller

Mix 1 T. of cornstarch with water or milk and drink it. Mrs Ruben Schwartz

For diarrhea relief, take 1/4 tsp. cinnamon to a cup of warm water. Take this mixture 3 to 4 times a day until symptoms are relieved.

To get relief from diarrhea, try eating a lot of applesauce. Another option is to drink blackberry juice. You can drink up to 3 cups every several hours, or as needed.
Mrs. Edward Hertzler

According to numerous scientific studies, honey kills the bacteria that causes diarrhea.. So when you're plagued, take honey in tea or teaspoons.

1 qt. water	4 T. sugar	3/4 cup Tang
1 tsp. baking soda	1/4 tsp. salt	

Mix the above ingredients together well and store in the refrigerator. This should be used up in a few days.   David & Treva Lambright

For diarrhea or upset stomach, squeeze the juice out of 2 lemons and add them to a quart of warm water, but don't add sugar. Drink a cupful at a time until empty. This usually settles the stomach quickly.   Mrs. Levi S. Miller

Steam carrots for 10 minutes not longer and do not boil then mash them and juice it if there is any and give to children for diarrhea, also works for diarrhea in calves.   Junior Miller

DIURETIC TEA

1 marigold flower (pick fresh every day)   6 chicory flowers
2 plantain leaves 6 red clover blossoms   1 Comfrey leaf
Steep the above ingredients in 1 qt. of boiling water for 15 minutes. Do not boil the herbs. For variation and flavor add mint, lemon balm, catnip, or anything else you desire. This is a good tea to aid in digestion and kidney function.

Mrs. Moses Z. Stoltzfus

A good mess of dandelion greens made into a warm salad is a wonderful spring tonic and is good for kidney problems. Because dandelion greens and dried powdered dandelion roots are one of the best diuretics known. Dandelion is also good for diabetics.

Atlee E Miller

DIABETES SORES

Make a paste of lard and flour and put it directly on the sores. It worked very well for sores from diabetes.

Esther Otto

DIZZINESS

Dizziness can be relieved by drinking a glass of water with a splash of vinegar added to it.

Atlee E Miller

DROPSY/EDEMA/FLUID RETENTION

Dropsy consists of an accumulation of fluid in the body tissues. It will cause death from internal drowning if severe enough. Dropsy is a vast accumulation of toxic wastes in liquid form. If they aren't eliminated from the body fast enough, they are deposited in any available space throughout our body's cells and gradually dehydrated and crystallized. This continues until a saturation point is reached and then nature will reverse the process by slowly dissolving the crystalized and dehydrated material. This change is the body's effort to save the life from being snuffed out caused by complete stoppage. The body eliminates toxins through our breathing, the skin, the colon, the kidneys, and the sinuses in this order. Our eliminative organs become overworked and clogged, especially the kidneys, liver and heart, slowing down the elimination process yet more. The body then steadily increases in size until it can no longer sustain life.

Start on the lemon juice diet (see Body Cleanse I). Drink several glasses of hot lemonade with cayenne pepper (drink prepared in lemon juice diet) before each session. Obtain about 100# or so of coarse rock salt from a feed store. Cover the bottom of an empty bathtub with about 2" of salt. Unclothe and wrap yourself in a wet sheet. Lay in the tub on the salt. Surround yourself completely with at least 2" of salt. Lay in this salt for one hour. Retrieve the salt and store for the next use. Take a bath or shower. Repeat every day or every other day for up to thirty days or until a big change takes place. The first time, not much change will be noticed, but from then on a noticeable change should take place.

For fluid-retention problems, take 2 vitamin B-6 tablets before every meal. You can also try 1 T. of lemon juice that comes in a bottle mixed with a glass of water both in the morning and the evening.

Mrs. Andy H. Miller

Drinking one cup of horsetail tea a day will help keep the retention of fluid down.

Lizzie Yoder

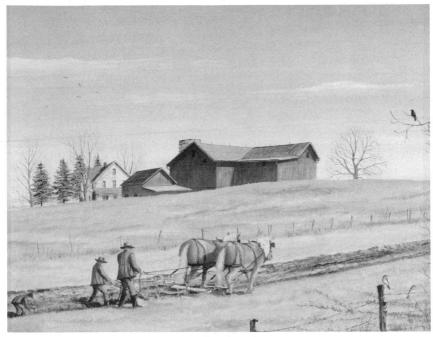

Plowing

This is an old recipe from a doctor for what they used to call dropsy. Take the bark off of wild grape vines and dry it. Burn it and use the ashes. The proportions should be 1 tsp. with 4 oz. red grape wine - it must be red.

4 oz. grape juice   4 oz. water
1 rounded tsp. cream of tartar   1 lemon
Take this 4 times a day for 5 days.   Amos Miller

Another remedy is to take 1 tsp. cream of tartar with the juice of one lemon and 4 oz. of red grape wine. Use this 3 times a day for 1 week. This can be used with water if it's too strong. (See also Diuretic Tea)   Amos Miller

DROWSINESS
Deeply inhale the aroma from a sliced garlic clove.

Take 3 ginseng capsules before you leave for church. This will help you listen to the sermon with your eyes open. This should not be done right before bedtime.
                                            Mrs Levi S Miller

EAR CARE
Boil the infected ear out with peroxide then put in drops of garlic oil. Cover the ear with a warm cloth if possible.   Mrs. Andy Keim

Place a drop of warmed (not hot) vinegar in the sore ear.   Perry J Miller

45

To dissolve excess ear wax, put 1/4 teaspoon of baking soda in 1 oz. of warm water. Store in a small dropper bottle and put 3 drops in the ear 3 times a day for 5-7 days. This will soften the wax and make it easily flushed out with a bulb syringe. To do an immediate flush, mix 1 teaspoon baking soda and 1 teaspoon Epsom Salt in 4 oz. of water and flush with a bulb syringe.

-DeVon Miller

Dip a cotton ball in peppermint oil and place in the affected ear.

Mrs Andy J Byler

To clear the infection from an ear, put 1/4 capful of peroxide into each ear. Lie flat, with the ear up and pull up on the earlobe. You can feel the peroxide drain down deep in the ear. It will foam and get warm. Sit up and let it drain out, then repeat this treatment for the other ear. I often repeat this two times for the first treatment. On the first day do this three times - morning, noon, and night. This will take about 4 - 5 days to clear.

For earache relief put some olive oil on cotton and then add some black pepper. Rub this on the outside of the ear. Do not put inside the ear.

Melvin & Inez Mullet

A surefire method of preventing earaches and plugged ears is to take a 1 tsp. of Swedish Bitters in water or juice before going to bed every night. I had constant problems with my ears before trying this remedy and now I'm not bothered at all with them either hurting or closing up.   Lydia Swarey

Wrap some onion slices in tin foil and put them on a broiler until juicy. Put the juice from the onions into the ear.   Wilbur & Wilma Miller

For ear infections, nothing works better than garlic extract. You can use this in either capsule form or liquid. You put it in the ear 3 times a day.

Susan Yoder

Cut garlic cloves into fine pieces and cover with olive oil. Let this set for 3 - 4 days and then drain off the oil. I add 1 oz. of tea tree oil to about 16 oz. of garlic oil.

Mrs Joseph W. Schrock

Put equal parts of vinegar and alcohol together. Put a drop or so of this in the ear. This also works for inner ear infections.   Anna M. Miller

Cut a raw potato in half and finely shred out the heart of it. Put it on a soft tissue and warm it. Put it on the ear and cover with warm blanket. It gives immediate relief.   Mary Detweiler

To relieve itchy ears, try mixing 1 T. vinegar with 3 T. water. Dip a cotton swab in this solution to clean your ears. It works very well.   Sam E Miller

Put room-temperature peroxide in ear several times a week, to remove initial build up of ear wax. Then continue to use once a month regularly. For itchy ears, soak a Q-tip in peroxide and rub it around inside the ear.   Annie J Peachey

Swimmers can reduce their chances of developing ear infections by using vinegar ear drops. Dilute vinegar half and half with water and use after every session.

Rebecca Miller

Swimmers who have problems with ear infection, should wear ear plugs when swimming.

For earache put 1-2 drops kyolic liquid - aged garlic extract in ear every four hours. These has also been use to cure ear infection if used every hour.

William Beachy

For earache, open a soft gel garlic and put oil right in ear. Works excellent.

Amos Yoder

EYE CARE
For a sty or infected eye, put a wooden spoon in boiling water until the spoon is hot. Wrap the spoon in a cloth and hold it on the infected eye. Do this several times a day until the infection or sty is gone.   Irene Yoder

For any eye infection use Rosebud Salve to rub the eye with.

To remove an object from the eye, put a flax seed in the affected eye. The dust, etc. will disappear and the flax seed will remove itself.   Jacob Christner

Mineral water makes a great face freshener. Just fill a spray bottle with chilled mineral water and "mist" your freshly-washed face with it. The mineral water plumps your skin and invigorates you just as well as more expensive, bottled or canned waters would at only a fraction of the cost.   Noah J Petersheim

For helping eyes get back to normal use honey. Just put a drop or so in the eyes. It will burn like fire at first but only for a few seconds. (my eyes improved) I was just ready to get glasses. My eyes had been dry.   Rebecca Miller

For cataracts in eyes, use better than half of honey and Heinz Vinegar, put a few drops in eyes, it hurts but saves money.   Amos Miller

For sore eyes in babies or children, put a little boric acid in warm water and use cotton balls dipped in the water and wash their eyes with it, a couple times a day.

FERTILITY
Eating garlic regularly in your diet will increase fertility. It is an aphrodisiac and is a libido stimulant. (see also Health Maintenance)

Editor's Note: A 100 years ago, people who were infertile went on the bear fat diet. We were unable to locate this diet as of press time but believe it to be very valuable information. We would like to locate this if it is to be found yet. From what we've been reading and hearing about infertility, the causes have more to do with the overall toxic condition of the body rather than some special isolated single thing you can do or take. (See Body Cleanse I)

FEVER

Use chopped raw onions on the soles of the feet overnight for fevers. Wear tight socks to keep the onions in place. For babies and small children, a thin layer of cloth may be put between the onions and the skin to keep from blistering.

Mrs Eli Bontrager

To rid your child of a fever, bathe them in strong, warm vinegar water. You may add a little dry mustard if you so desire.

Fannie J Stutzman

Beat the white of an egg and drink it down. This should take the fever away or at least give some relief.

Milton & Lizzie J Yoder

To break a fever or check a cold in the early stages, mix 2 T. of lemon and honey mixture to a cup of water. Children like this and almost never fails.

Rub vinegar on the forehead, temples, palms of your hands, and bottoms of your feet to get rid of a fever. Repeat as needed every 20 - 25 minutes.

Melvin & Inez Mullet

Take a dab of sugar (1/8 tsp.) and a dab of cream of tartar (1/8 tsp.) and fill the rest of the tsp. with water. Take this every 15 minutes until the fever breaks.

Mrs Wanda Bontrager

For fever relief, soak your socks in vinegar and then put them on. They will soon dry. It draws the fever out. For small children, dilute the vinegar with water.

John J Burkholder

Vinegar is very good for bringing down a fever. Soak a pair of wool socks in pure vinegar and put them on the fevered person's feet. Put a dry pair of warmed wool socks over the top of the wet ones. Keep the feet warm. My mother always said the feet should be warm for this treatment.

Mrs. Lloyd Kuepfer

I use vinegar for fever. Wipe in their hands, on soles of feet, on top of back. Put on a warm vinegar rag, then put a warm towel on. Do this as often as you wish.

Dan S Swartzentruber

To rid someone of a fever, slice onions about 1/2" thick and put the slices in their socks before putting the socks on. Leave the onion slices there over night and the fever will be gone in the morning. Eating onions also works as a natural antibiotic

Mrs. Glen H Lambright

If you have fever and feel sick all over bathe your feet in hot vinegar water. This can often make you feel lots better.

Alvin Yoder

Put a wet vinegar rag on the breast, change off every time the rag feels warm will drive fever out fast. It also works on the feet if fever isn't too high.

Daniel A Hershberger

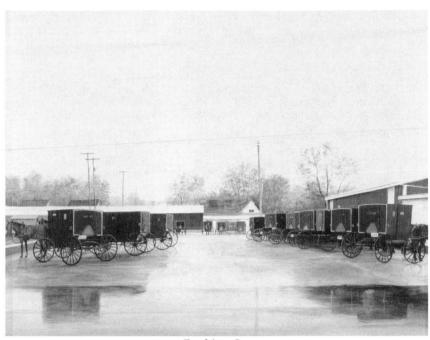

Parking Lot

FLU
If you have the flu or a bad cold take 1/2 cup of homemade wine and add 1 teaspoon of ginger to it and warm till lukewarm. Drink it and go to bed and sweat. You will be feeling somewhat better by morning. This was used by our grandparents. Pete & Mary Eicher

To the person with chills, try using capsicum (or red pepper) capsules. Try 1 or 2 a day with a cup of milk. You could also try soaking your feet in a pail full of water as hot as you can stand it, with a cup or 2 of vinegar added to it. Soak your feet until the water cools off, then add more hot water and repeat the process. Never walk on cold floors without shoes on and always sleep with pajamas and socks on. Lizzie Yoder

Put some vinegar in your bath water and soak for awhile. Mrs Jacob L Miller

Tea made of ginger a little honey and hot water is good for the flu. Makes the stomach feel so good. Lloyd Kuepfer

Fight flu fast with garlic salve. Coat the soles of your feet with olive oil then rub a sliced garlic clove on them. Cover them with socks. Go to bed and wake up feeling like a new person. John S Eicher

If you get a head flu take a glass of water and put some apple cider vinegar in the glass of water then add a tablespoon of soda in the vinegar water and drink it when it is still foaming. That clears your head. John S Eicher

1 T. soda in a glass of water for 3 days, never more then 3 days, the body would become too alkaline. The body is an acid state when flu strikes. Take once or twice daily.   Simon S Schwartz

FOOD POISONING
When traveling, always take a bottle of apple cider vinegar along. When you have to eat in a questionable restaurant, drink 1 tsp. of apple cider vinegar in a glass of water to prevent food poisoning. This is helpful if taken every five minutes in case of food poisoning. Garlic will also work.   Barbara Miller

For food poisoning swallow raw egg whites until you feel better. This has been tried with good results.   Katie Miller

1 T. of apple juice vinegar in glass of water. Can repeat dose in 2 to 3 hours.
                                                                       Simon S Schwartz

For food poisoning eat dry bread. I saw very good results with this.
                                                                    Gideon E Gingerich

FOOT CARE
Get rid of corns and bunions by bandaging them overnight with slices of raw onion and old bread wetted down with lots of full-strength vinegar. End foot odors by soaking the feet a couple of times a week in 1/3 cup vinegar, added to a small pan of water. Toss in one tea bag also.   Mrs. Mattie Ann Miller

To keep your feet from perspiring so much, bathe them in very warm water for 30 minutes twice a week. A little salt or Epsom salt may be added. Add 1 tsp. of boric acid to 1 quart of hot water. Soak for at least 20 minutes or more.
                                                                   Herman D Gingerich

Rub apple cider vinegar over them (especially between the toes) after every washing.   Mary E Beachy

Sprinkle baking soda in your shoes to get rid of foot odor.   Johnny Miller

FROSTBITE
1 oz. olive oil 1 oz. turpentine 1 oz. peppermint oil 1 oz. ammonia
Mix the above ingredients and put in a bottle. Apply a small amount to the frost-bitten area and rub in well.   Mrs. Atlee N. Troyer

GALL STONES
Try drinking only juices (no food) for 1 whole day. In the evening take 6 oz. of olive oil followed by pure lemon juice. The next morning take a small dose of Epsom salt or any other good laxative. You will expel the stones without pain. They'll be green and easily identified.   Jacob Christner

Drink 1 qt. pure apple juice between meals for 3 days and, on the evening of the third day, take 4 oz. of cold pressed olive oil mixed with grapefruit juice. Don't eat supper on the third day and don't eat solids right away the next morning.
                                                                          Ida C Miller

Take the juice of 3 lemons, 3 tsp. cream of tartar, and 3 tsp. of Epsom Salts, and put them in a pint jar. Fill the jar with water, stirring the mixture up every morning. Take 1 T. every morning before breakfast. Comfrey root tea is also good for gall bladder trouble, along with stomach ailments, liver problems and kidney stones. (See also Body Cleanse)   Mrs. Andy H. Miller

HAIR CARE
This is a remedy I use when washing my hair. I either use vinegar on the hair and rub it in or put some vinegar in the water when rinsing my hair.   Amos Miller

Soak your hair with apple cider vinegar for one hour before washing. Repeat, if necessary.   Judy Mast

Add a pinch of borax to the water that you use to wash your hair.
                                                Mary S Yoder

To get rid of dandruff, take some strong sage tea and a little soap to wash your head, then rinse very well with a little vinegar in the rinse water.
                                            Fannie J Stutzman

One teaspoon vinegar in one cup of water is a great final rinse for the hair. It is a preventive against dandruff or scaling of the scalp.
                                              Atlee E Miller

Put a few drops of Tea Tree Oil into your shampoo bottles to get rid of dandruff and for a good feeling scalp.   Mabel Miller

For thicker hair growth, rub some peach leaf tea onto your scalp. Your hair growth should become healthier.   Lydia Petersheim

To make your hair more manageable after washing, add vinegar to the rinse water.   Enos R Byler

Put several drops of baby oil in the rinse water. It makes your hair healthier and more manageable.   Jacob Christner

If you have a problem with an itchy scalp, use vinegar in your rinse water when washing your hair.   William Miller

Use a bit of vinegar in the final rinse water to take the frizz out of a new permanent and to revive and old one.   Rebecca Miller

A full head of healthy, richly colored hair can be ensured, well into old age, you need only to start each day water to which has been added 4 teaspoons each of apple cider vinegar, black strap molasses, and honey. Sylvia L Shetler

HEADACHE
Drink the juice of one lemon with a cup of warm water, and repeat this every 15 minutes.   Mrs. Levi S Miller

For headache relief use a hot, wet vinegar cloth over the head.

Mrs. Jacob L. Miller

Taking a hot foot bath in water to which 2 tsp. of powdered mustard have been added can relieve headaches. While soaking the feet for 20 to 30 minutes, apply a folded handkerchief that has been dampened with equal parts of cold water and vinegar, to the head. Re-dampen the handkerchief frequently.   Mary S. Yoder

Feverfew, a healing herb, has been prized for relief of migraine headaches since the the the time of the Roman Empire. It is believed to reduce the pain in the head by influencing the way blood vessels contract. Do not use at the same time as other pain relievers such as aspirin or warfarin.

Two teaspoons of honey with each meal will banish migraine headaches. If you feel one coming on. A quick teaspoon can help. Or boil equal parts of vinegar and honey and inhale the steam.   Atlee E Miller

To rid yourself of migraines, take 2 tsp. of honey with each meal. If you feel a migraine coming on, a quick tsp. can help a lot. Another remedy is to boil equal parts of vinegar and honey and inhale the steam.   Mrs. Mattie Ann Miller

HEAD LICE
For killing head lice, use regular mouth wash 2-3 times, 7 days apart to wash your hair. It is important to comb out the nits (lice eggs) with a fine toothed comb. Clean and desanitize the floors, furniture, and bedding of your house at the same times to prevent reinfestation from hatchlings. Use coconut shampoo to wash your hair with to help repel them. Head lice can't stand the smell.   Mabel Miller

For head lice use camphorated oil. Cover the entire hair area with it and put something over the hair for overnight. Shampoo the oil out as you usually would the next morning.   Mrs. Andy J Byler

The best treatment for head lice is to cover the head with mayonnaise and then cover the head with Saran wrap for a while. It's a messy treatment, but it kills all the lice.   Mrs Clarence Miller

If there would be a lice epidemic in your community, rub "oil of sassafras" behind ears for a preventative. They can't stand the smell.   Raymond Schwartz

To get rid of head-lice use (rubbing) Alcohol instead of the expensive things from the drug store. Use 2 or 3 times the same as the other, but you want to lie down as it is suffocating if you hang your hair over your face. We had better luck with this.   Wilmer E Schrock

HEALTH MAINTENANCE
An ancient Greek physician once said, "Let food be your medicine, and medicine your food." It is still good advice today. Some experts say today that the most effective cures can be found right in your kitchen cabinet. One of Rome's most renowned physicians often recommended garlic. During the Middle Ages a heavy dose of mustard was used for various respiratory ailments. Modern pharma-

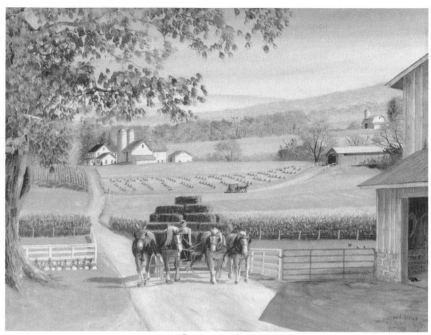

Summertime

cologists turned to chemicals for developing medications, mostly because their formulations could be protected by a patent, thus protecting their incomes. Not so with the natural remedies. As a result, the natural ways were almost buried and forgotten. Today, a growing number of people, fearful of the long term side effects of modern medicine and discouraged by high health costs, are turning back to the old natural ways.

The three pillars of most all the old remedies were garlic, honey and apple cider vinegar. These 3 used in combination are often stronger and more effective when used together. They have a long rich history as natural remedies for many different ailments. Natural healers have known this for centuries, but many of these cures were denounced as old wives fables. This is a serious mistake. There is no question that modern medicine has been a lifesaver, but sometimes the old ways are the best ways. Garlic especially has been lauded as one of the most effective herbal treatments known to man, a wonder drug.It was prescribed by Pliny the Elder, a renowned Roman naturalist, as the cure for over 60 different medical disorders. Modern scientists proved in lab tests what naturalists have known for centuries; that garlic is a wonder medicine, a natural antibiotic with no side effects. It kills pathogenic bacteria while supporting developement of the natural bacterial flora in the digestive tract. Studies show that garlic is the most effective when consumed fresh and raw. Cooking garlic destroys the phytochemical allicin which makes it so effective. The act of crushing the raw garlic clove by chewing or blending it, releases the herb's allicin. In Jean Carper's book, it is reported that Russian officials once sent 500 tons of garlic throughout the country to quash an outbreak of deadly influenza. Researchers mixed blood cells from people who had eaten lots of raw garlic and were stunned when 160% more cancer cells were killed when compared to the blood from people who hadn't eaten any garlic. Only one odorless garlic extract, Kyolic, has been proven to be as effective as raw garlic. For neutralizing the pungent odor of garlic breath, suggestions are honey, yogurt, cottage cheese, milk, red wine, or a snip of parsley. Honey and apple cider vinegar are simple inexpensive foods. Honey has a very impressive history as a healing remedy and vinegar is a well known antiseptic containing many disinfecting and healing properties. So keep plenty of these natural miracle foods in your kitchen cupboards. You'll be doing yourself and your family a favor, and saving a lot of money in the process.

JOHANNA'S MIX

3 bulb fresh garlic   4-5 T. raw honey

8 oz cottage cheese or yogurt

Grind together in a blender and store in the refridgerator in glass containers. The honey will help preserve the mix and then heal and cleanse you. The cottage cheese or yogurt will prevent your stomach from becoming sore from the garlic. (Editor's Note: This remedy was sent to us from Germany by the undersigned. By using this she recovered from heart disease, clots causing a stroke, a tumor on her brain and regained her mobility and memory. She continues to take some of this at least once every week for good maintenance.)   Johanna Runyan

MIRACLE TEA

2 tsp honey   2 tsp apple cider vinegar

Mix into a glass of regular (no caffiene) tea. This amazing tea is delicious and was used by doctors in the past for healing numerous ailments including allergies, baldness, brittle bones and nails, burns, chronic headaches, cold hands and feet, colds, flu, constipation, deafness, dizziness, fatigue, heart disease, hemorrhoids, hypertension, impotence, insomnia, poor memory, muscle tension, sore throat, and varicose veins. Sipping just 2 teaspoons of miracle tea at each meal can produce a weight loss of up to 10 pounds a month. Brew a batch of tea and store it in a glass jar and keep in the refridgerator. This will make it convenient to add the honey and vinegar for taking it consistently. You can drink it or rub it on externally.

Dr Jarvis

Over the years many have used the old time honey and vinegar remedies which follow to promote good health, general well being, and environmentally safe cleaning. Many claims have been made for the daily consumption of a honey and vinegar tonic. The basic, time honored dose is two teaspoons of honey and two teaspoons of vinegar, stirred into a full glass of tepid water. When served with each meal, it seems to protect from the most distressing features of aging. Those who take this combination on a regular basis seem to feel young and vigorous well into their supposable 'twilight years.' Honey and vinegar are considered by many to be an almost magical combination for the treatment of sleeplessness. Stir a little vinegar into a cup of honey. Administer by the spoonful at bedtime, and again wherever needed in the night. It is a natural, time tested remedy for a vexing problem.   Rebecca Miller

Garlic is a natural antibiotic. We've had good results using it for things such as sore throats, flu, high blood pressure, etc. We use it just like penicillin. Take one clove

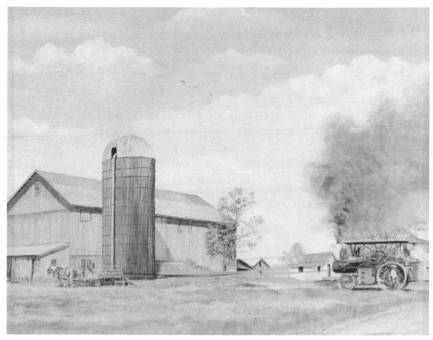

Steam Engine

(or two if very small) and cut it in pieces. You can swallow the pieces just like a pill. Take one piece 3 or 4 times a day until you feel better. You should see results in not more than 3 - 4 days, usually sooner. The key is to start using it before you become very sick. For babies and small children we make garlic oil by soaking grated garlic in pure virgin olive oil for 2 weeks, shaking occasionally. Pour the oil until the garlic is covered, but not much more. After 2 weeks drain and store the oil out of the sunlight. To neutralize garlic breath, eat a piece of parsley.

Mrs Ben Hershberger

Comfrey tea is good for a number of things. Some of these are - a blood cleanser in the spring, coughs, diarrhea, female debility, kidneys, stomach, bowels, bruises or pain. A broken arm or foot may even be soaked in the tea to speed up the healing process. A poultice of fresh leaves is real good for bee stings or any kind of insect bite or sting. It will take the poison out. Another option is to soak dried leaves in water and then put the wet leaves on the bite or sting. Katie Lehman

Tea made from Plantain (pigs ears) leaves is a good remedy for diarrhea, kidney and bladder trouble or infection, aching in the lumbar region and bed wetting. It's also wonderful for parasites. It will help clear the head of mucus and heals stings or snake bites, carbuncles and tumors. Anyone who has a "Back to Eden" book should look it up. It has been known to cure Bright's Disease and Nephritis when all medicines failed. It can also be given to babies with jaundice. The Indians used this weed to a great advantage. It is at it's prime to gather in late spring or early summer to dry it and use for tea.   Mrs Noah J Swartzentruber

Use 1 T. natural vinegar and 1 T. honey in a glass of warm water. Drink a glass of this first thing in the morning upon rising for a healthier you.

Amanda Hershberger

2 tsp. wheat germ   2 tsp. lecithin
1/4 tsp. bone meal   1 tsp. brewer's yeast
This is a chelation recipe to clean out your blood stream. Mix the ingredients in an 8 oz. glass of water or your favorite drink.   Mary Graber

4 1/2 gallon clover flowers   3 gallon warm water
1 pkg. yeast   12 1/2 lb. Granulated sugar
Let the above mixture stand for 3 days. Remove flowers from the liquid and let it stand for an additional week, then stir every morning and evening. Strain and bottle. Do not tighten the lids. After setting for 2 months, pour the liquid into other jugs. Do not shake it up, but keep the brown in the bottom out so it will stay nice and clear. Cork it tightly. This works as a great blood purifier.

Lizzie Yoder

When you feel yourself getting sick, drink more liquids like water, tea, etc. (at least 8 glasses per day). Slack off on eating food. Refrain especially from any food that has white sugar or white flour in it.   DeVon & Mabel Miller

We have been giving our children barley grass and colloidal silver for over a year, and they haven't been sick much all winter. Barley grass helps build up their immune system and silver helps fight infection. I wouldn't want to be without it!

John J Miller

Take Black Strap Molasses for improving your blood's ability to coagulate and heal all those cuts and bruises.   DeVon & Mabel Miller

Grind up, peelings and all, 6 lemons, 6 oranges, and 6 grapefruit. Add 4 T. of Epsom Salts and pour in 1 qt. of boiling water. Let this stand overnight. In the morning, put the mixture in a cloth bag and press out all the juice. Take 1 T. of this juice 3 times a day. Keep it in a cool place, to keep it from spoiling. This can also be made in 1/3 or 1/2 batches. Another good remedy is to use dandelion as a blood purifier.   Amanda A. Miller

Placing fresh mullein leaves in your shoes has been noted to draw poisons from your body. Make sure to use fresh leaves daily.

To get rid of toxins in your body, soak in a cider vinegar bath for 10-15 minutes, 2 times a week. This is a very clean feeling bath. Make sure you wipe your skin very well with a washcloth while soaking. This is also a good soaking treatment for most skin sores and even helps to open pores so that you can perspire more freely.   Emanuel Yoder Family

2 lg. T. honey   2 qt. water   3/4 cup apple cider vinegar
This can be made to taste. If using homemade vinegar, the acid content may vary.   Atlee Miller Family

For a tune up on your body, squeeze a whole lemon into a pint jar, and then fill the jar with water. Take a few swallows every so often throughout the day or until it's gone. Do this every day for a whole week.   Katie Miller

To help regulate bowel movements, drink a glass of warm water as soon as you get up and the last thing before going to bed at night. Drink at least eight glasses of water throughout the day.   Mrs Andy J Byler

Take 1 T. of pure cider vinegar and 1 T. of honey in a glass of water. Mix well and take this every meal, especially when waking every morning. This is good for aches and pains in the lower back, dizziness, dull headaches, dull hair, unmanageable hair, bloodshot eyes, tired eyes, extreme loss of mental alertness, nervousness, depression, cold hands and feet. All of these ailments can be caused by low potassium and cider vinegar and honey are high in potassium.   Annie Petersheim

A very good remedy for liver, kidneys, colon, and numerous other thing, such as being filled with drugs etc. Start in the morning at 6:00 and drink 4 oz. distilled water every 1/2 hour. (Distilled means boiled, I boil mine usually for 20 minutes. At 12:00 noon you must rest or lay down and close your eyes, no writing, no reading, or anything. At 1:00 get up again and resume your drinking until 6.00. Do this every day for one month. Eat, drink, and chew anything else, but keep up with the water. It is surprising what all works out. This is very good to flush the sore and sensitive stomach flush the colon, rinse out kidneys and liver and cleanse the blood system. If trying to wash drugs from the body , discontinue them or the water will be to no avail. Also helps numerous other things. It also helps low blood sugar. (It has to be distilled water.) A gallon of water is plenty for one day.   Mosie J Shetler

Use blackstrap molasses (or the pills) to keep from getting constipated. It will also help make your menstrual cycle easier, if taken regularly.   B Yoder

Take a little Epsom Salt under your tongue every morning before you eat. Will prevent various diseases, and you'll have more accurate bowel movements. My dad had a broken bone. The doctor said he'll have a slow recovery. So he took a little Epsom salt under his tongue every morning, and the doctor was really amazed how fast it healed.   Daniel A Hershberger

For natural well-being take garlic pills daily. You can get the odorless kind or you can raise your own, and eat a garlic bulb daily. If you eat a little parsley with this it takes care of the odor. Parsley can also be raised and dried. The garlic is good for numerous things. It's a natural antibiotic, takes care of parasites etc.
     Joseph W Bontreger

Two teaspoons apple cider vinegar in 1/2 glass of water two or three a day is good to drink to loose weight, heart burn, hay fever, kidney trouble, and lots of other ailments.   Ammon C Stutzman

For sluggish liver, colds, sinus, etc. Make a drink of, 1/2 lemon juice, 2 T. maple syrup, 1/8 to 1/4 tsp. cayenne pepper. Put all into a glass and fill with filtered cold water. Drink every morning for first thing.   Junior Detweiler

1 cup Apple Cider Vinegar, 1 cup Epsom Salt, 1 Tablespoon ground ginger, Put this in a bath tub of hot water (as hot as you can stand) as much as you can get in the tub. Soak till you start getting weak. Do this every day till you can stay in for 20 minutes. We've had really good results for flu, aching body, sluggishness, or anything else that we encountered. As this pulls toxins out of the body. A few times when I was pretty sick and did this I felt really weak. So maybe wouldn't want to be alone. It makes one really sweat and then you want to go directly to bed and not get cold.   Wilmer E Schrock

The way to stay healthy and alert, well into old age, is to combine one teaspoon of vinegar, one teaspoon of honey, and a full glass of water. Take this tonic three times a day, 1/2 hour before meals.   Sylvia L Shetler

Red and white clover blossom tea is a splendid blood purifier.
                                                        Mrs Eli L Glick

HEART ATTACKS/STROKES
For heart attacks or strokes, squirt cayenne extract or tincture under the tongue several times. Or put a teaspoon of cayenne pepper in a glass of warm water and have the victim drink it or take a dropper and put under the tongue. We know it works! After Dad was home several days from the hospital after being there for pneumonia and a light heart attack, he had severe chest pains. My husband put several squirts of cayenne tincture under the tongue and a little while later no severe pains anymore.   Clyde Yoder

HEAT RASH
You can put either lemon juice or vinegar in your bath water. This will help to neutralize acid on the skin. Also, you can put baking soda on the rash with good results.   Judy Mast

HEMORRHOIDS
Insert one garlic clove several inches into the rectum and leave it there. When it is expelled with a bowel movement, insert another one. This has gotten rid of hemorrhoids so that they never return.   Lena Yoder

Take 1 T. of blackstrap molasses before breakfast followed by a glass of water. Within weeks you should see good results.   Mrs. Andy H. Miller

Mix 1/2 teaspoon of mild mustard powder with 1 T. of raw honey and apply it with a cotton swab.

HICCUPS
Take 1 T. of Damson Plum Jelly to cure your hiccups.

To get relief from hiccups, eat a tsp. of peanut butter. It works very well.
                                                        Sam E Miller

Take a long drink of water.

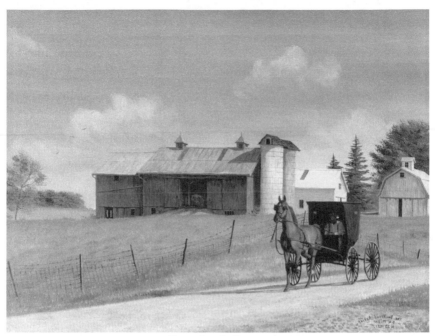

Grandpa's Buggy

HIVES
For hives, use liquid chlorophyll diluted in water. The hives usually disappear in a half day or so.   Mrs Andy Keim

Give some cream of tartar and sulfur in a half/half measurement. Take a dab 3 times a day before meals.   Mrs J Λ Hershberger

HOT FLASHES
Detoxify the liver to get rid of hot flashes by taking the juice of a half lemon and add it to 3 - 4 oz. of water. Take this first thing in the morning. Mrs. Andy Keim

Native Americans have long used Black Cohosh to treat women's gynecological ailments. It can be just as effective as estrogen in treating the sudden sweats and "gloomies" associated with menopause. It is both safe and effective to use.

INDIGESTION
Vinegar or garlic is a good remedy to take before going to bed after consuming greasy foods. Take 2 T. with water.   Amos Miller

Mix 1 teaspoon honey and 1 teaspoon apple cider vinegar in a glass of warm water and drink it 1/2 hour before you eat.

If you have heartburn, indigestion (bloating), or want to maintain good overall health, try eating a walnut size raw red potato every day.

For indigestion put 1 tsp. caraway seeds in a cup of hot water, let it cool and drink it.   Amos Miller

INSECT STINGS
What child hasn't been stung of a bee or wasp at one time or another? To ease the pain, mix a teaspoon of unseasoned meat tenderizer with a few drops of water to make a paste then place this on the injury. This will give your child almost instantaneous relief since an enzyme in meat tenderizer dissolves the toxins that the insect has injected with its stinger. A similar application of baking soda is a good second choice. Remove the stinger by carefully lifting it up with a clean fingernail or blade of some type then scraping gently. John S Eicher

To heal a bee sting, put some vinegar and baking soda on the bite to keep the swelling down. It must be done immediately to be effective.   Mrs. Toby H. Yoder

For relief of bee stings, get a plantain (pig ear) leaf. Rub the leaf on the sting until it quits hurting. These leaves can sometimes be found in your own yard.

After an insect bite or sting, immediately rub some hand soap onto the area before it swells. Place half an onion on the sting until it is gone.

For relief of bee stings, get a plantain or peach tree leaf and tape it directly on the area of the bee sting. It will stop hurting directly.   Mary S Yoder

To ease the sting of those summertime pests, put full strength vinegar on the affected area. Another option is to make a paste of baking soda and water and put it on the affected area. Try treating the area with a piece of cotton soaked with vinegar.   Milton & Lizzie J Yoder

For bees, wasps, or bumblebee stings put soda on a spoon then add pure vinegar to make a paste. Put this on the sting and it here will soon be less pain.
                                                             Elmer Yoder

Fill a tablespoon half full with cider vinegar, add a half tsp. soda or enough so it's still good and moist. Put on bee sting repeatedly for instant relief. apply while it sizzles.   Alvin Yoder & Jacob Stutzman & John Stutzman

Mix tenderquick with vinegar to make a paste for insect bites. Apply immediately.   William Beachy

INSOMNIA
If you have trouble sleeping, try putting a hot water bottle on your stomach when you go to bed.   Lydia Petersheim

If you're unable to sleep, drink a cup of hot milk, take a teaspoon of honey or take calcium 30 minutes to 1 hour before going to bed.   Mrs Andy J Byler

Sleeplessness and mild depression can often be helped with St Johns Wart.
                                                             William Beachy

INTESTINAL DISTRESS
Apple cider vinegar has no side affects and can prevent intestinal distress, which can have serious health consequences. Vinegar attacks bacteria as well as other harmful intestinal parasites. You will notice a less unpleasant smell of the stool within a few days. A foul smelling stool is an indication that something is wrong.   Barbara Miller

Take a cup of raw oatmeal and 3 cups of water. Let soak several minutes and pour off the water. Give this to the child. If your child is still using a bottle, give this remedy instead of milk. This water is also good for eczema or diaper rash. Just rub it on.   Mrs. Harley Miller

ITCHING
Mince 6 garlic cloves and steep them in hot, just boiled water for 20 minutes, then strain. Adding vitamin E will encourage quick healing. Rub this over the affected area.

Itchy skin can be relieved by substituting one teaspoon of vinegar in 1/2 glass of water for the usual soap one may be using. Simply rub this potion into the skin and forgo the irritation of soap.   Rebecca Miller

Spray area with diluted apple cider vinegar, being careful to stay off the sensitive area.   Mary E Beachy

For itchiness and spots over body, discontinue using fabric softener and use Apple Cider Vinegar instead. Also bath in vinegar water. Some itchiness and spots can also come from liver not working properly. Vinegar will also soften your wash.
                                                    Mosie J Shetler

JAUNDICE
Take 1 heaping T. of crushed peach leaves to a cup of boiling water. Cover this and strain. When it becomes cool enough to drink, take 4 cups a day.

KIDNEY/BLADDER INFECTIONS
For sluggish kidneys and/or bladder drink a tea made of parsley. You can add some mint tea for flavor. This is a sure cure.   Mrs. Glen H. Lambright

I've had several surgical procedures to rid myself of kidney stones and have tried other medical interventions without success. This home remedy has been more successful for me. I eat a lot of watermelon and sit in a hot tub to get my blood circulating. I also take 2 Magnesium tablets, and 2 B-6 tablets daily. I start with 2 of each every hour for one day. They seem to help break the stones down so I can pass them on my own more easily. Drinking a lot of water is also very important. Some teas work well, too. Some teas to drink are corn silk, watercress, uva ursi and juniper. Drink about a quart of one of these teas every day. If you're able, it also helps to take 2 T. of olive oil every 4 hours until the stones pass.
                                                    Amanda Helmuth

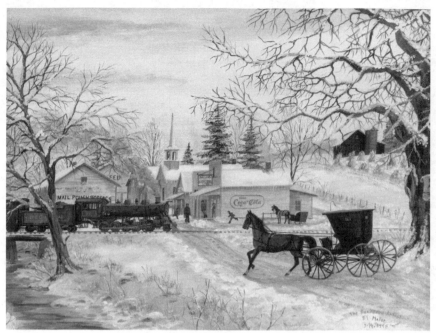

Train

Wash six ordinary size red beets. Do not slice them. In 3 quarts of water, boil them slowly so as not to boil the water away. After an hour, strain the water and bottle it, placing it in the ice box to prevent souring. Drink 3 glasses of this a day. The drink simply dissolves the stones, and you don't even pass them.

Mrs Lloyd Kuepfer

For kidney stones and bladder 3 T. lemon juice, 3 T. cream of tarter, 3 T. Epsom salt. Put in a pint jar and fill with water. Stir every morning and take 1 T. every morning before breakfast. Take as soon as stirred as settles quickly.

Amos Yoder

Put a few grains of alum (no more) and 1 T. lemon juice in half a glass of water. Usually one dose of this will do the trick to relieve the pain. Another solution is to make a tea of corn silk and/or parsley and drink it. For urinary tract or kidney infections, taking cranberry juice or cranberry pills regularly will help a great deal.

Annie J Peachey

A few good splashes of vinegar in a tall glass of water takes care of kidney, bladder and urinary tract infections. Drink as many glassfuls as you can for at least 2 days.

Mrs Andy Keim

For kidney infections or painful urination, drink 3 or 4 glasses of cranberry juice a day. You can drink more or less depending on how bad the pain is. If cranberry juice is not easy to get, try some cranberry sauce. You empty a small can of sauce into a jar and mix it well with water. This can be used the same as cranberry juice.

Drink plenty of saffron tea until symptoms are relieved. This is a tea made from flowers. Drink cranberry juice. Drinking parsley tea is also good.

For kidney problems put 1 T of vinegar in 1 glass of fresh water. Drink as needed. I had very good results with this.   Gideon E Gingerich & Rebecca Miller

Eating raw garlic has been proven to kill bacteria causing bladder infections.

For bladder infection, drink lots of cranberry juice. I have used cranberry sauce and mixed it with a quart or so of water, if I didn't have the juice on hand. Drink 3 or 4 glasses a day.

An excellent source of natural extracts, herbs, prepackaged bowel, liver, and kidney detox kits that give you the most bang for your buck is the American Botanical Society - Dr Richard Schultz PO Box 9699 Marina del Rey, CA 90295 www.herbdoc.com 800-437-2362

LAXATIVE
1 pt. hot water   2 T. Epsom salts   1/2 T. cream of tartar
Drink the above mixture first thing in the morning. Use as needed.
                                             Annie J. Peachey

For laxative take one pinch of Epsom salt for 3 days. I had very good results with this.   Gideon E Gingerich

LOW BLOOD SUGAR
We've had good results in using extra virgin olive oil for low blood sugar. The dosage should be 1 tsp. a day after a meal. If you take this on an empty stomach, it works as a laxative also. If taken with a meal, it will help regulate your bowels.
                                             Emanuel Yoder Family

MEMORY
Garlic can keep your mental edge sharp. Eat 1-3 cloves of garlic each day dipped in honey or chocolate.

Memory can be greatly improved by drinking a glass of warm water before each meal, with a teaspoon of apple cider vinegar stirred in.   Sylvia L Shetler

MENOPAUSE PROBLEMS
You may be able to reduce the severity of menopausal symptoms with the following vitamins and minerals: 300 - 500 mg. of magnesium, 500 - 1000 mg. of calcium, 800 IU of Vitamin E (400 IU twice a day). Take a multivitamin/mineral supplement that contains at least 100 percent of the six important B vitamins (thiamin, riboflavin, niacin, vitamin B6, vitamin B12 and pantothenic acid). You also might want to use an evening primrose oil supplement. See also "Hot Flashes, Blackstrap Molasses"   Dan A Wengerd

MENSTRUAL CRAMPS

For painful menstrual cramps, drink camp bark tea. To make the tea, place 4 T. of camp bark, 1 T. of pennyroyal and 1 - 2 tsp. of freshly grated ginger in a pot and add a quart of cold water. Slowly bring the water to a simmer. Cover the pot and let it simmer for 2 - 3 minutes. Then remove the tea from the heat, and let it steep for 30 minutes, then strain. Drink 1/4 cup every 15 minutes until cramping stops.   Dan A Wengerd

To alleviate menstrual cramps, take oregano in liberal amounts for a few days.

MONO

"My daughter had mono and recovered before the week was up." For one week take these every two hours around the clock: Vitamins B2, B5, B6, and C. Take a B complex twice a day. Drink a protein supplement between meals twice a day. The secret is to keep a steady stream of B vitamins in the system for one week.
                                        Nancy Turner Ft Worth, TX

MOTION SICKNESS

For motion sickness, take 2-3 ginger root capsules before meal on empty stomach, chewing 3-4 papaya enzyme tablets with meal also helps, before going away.
                                        Levi Weaver

MORNING SICKNESS

A good remedy for morning sickness is to take B-6 vitamins every morning. This may not work for everyone, but it was recommended by a midwife. I had really good results.   Mrs. Edward Hertzler

MOUTHWASH

A homemade mouthwash is simple to make. Use 1 tsp. salt and 1 tsp. baking soda in a 1/2 cup of water; rinse and gargle as needed. A drop of peppermint extract can be added for a minty taste.   Daniel L Miller

MUSCLE ACHES

Try rubbing areas with castor oil.   Ervin A Bontrager

For relief from those sore muscles, try rubbing olive oil into the sore areas before going to bed.

To keep those leg cramps away, take Vitamin E before going to bed.
                                        Mrs. Andy J. Byler

Prevent leg cramps by combining 1 tsp. honey, 1 tsp. apple cider vinegar and 1 T. calcium lactate in a 1/2 glass of water. This should be taken once a day.
                                        Mrs. Menno Steury

Fill your bathtub with as hot water as you can stand and add 1 cup vinegar and 1 cup Epsom Salts. Soak for awhile.   Mrs. Wanda Bontrager

If you have tired and aching feet put a 1/2 cup of apple cider vinegar in a tub of warm water and soak for 30 minutes.   Mrs. Andy J. Byler

Lay flat on your back and raise the right leg as far as it will go, letting your knee bend. Keep the left leg and back straight. Hold this position for six seconds, then relax. Do this three times on each leg. Repeat as often as you like. This exercise will wake up lazy muscles. It works best in the morning before you are tired from a long day.   Annie J Peachey

Add vinegar to your bathtub for a refreshing bath for babies and adults alike. This is much better than bubble bath.   Melvin & Sara Miller

For sore or aching backs or hips, use a hand towel soaked lightly in vinegar. Put this directly on the back and lie on a hot water bottle for 10 - 15 minutes.
                                           Emanuel Nisley

Rub sore muscles with vinegar. Will diminish soreness etc.
                                           Daniel A Hershberger

We put 1 cup vinegar, 1/2 cup Epsom salt, 1 T. 30% peroxide, and a little squirt liquid Dreft to our bath water. It relaxes muscles and really provides a soothing bathe.   Daniel A Hershberger

To loosen muscles add Epsom salt 4 cups to bath water. Keep adding hot water. Make as hot as you can stand   Rebecca Miller

If you feel like you're coming down with the flu or have very sore muscles soak in a tub of hot water with apple cider vinegar added 1 or 2 cups.
                                           Joseph W Bontreger

Prevent leg cramps by combining one teaspoon apple cider vinegar, and one tablespoon calcium lactate in 1/2 glass of water. This is taken once a day.
                                           Sylvia L Shetler

Cure twitches and reoccurring muscle cramps in one week by taking two teaspoons of honey with meals.   Rebecca Miller

To make a soothing bath, add 1/2 cup apple cider vinegar, 1/3 cup salt and two tablespoons sage to a tub of very warm water.   Rebecca Miller

Homemade vinegar hot patch works wonders. Make equal parts of water and vinegar. Soak a towel in the mix wring it out and apply to sore areas for 5 minutes. Then follow with a cold compress.   John S Eicher

NERVOUSNESS
For anyone who is restless, nervous and can't sleep, soak 1 tsp. of plain gelatin in 1 cup of cold water for 5 minutes and add 1 cup of boiling water. Stir until dissolved. Put about 2 tsp. of this in each glass or bottle of milk, tea or whatever you drink for supper. It can even be put over food. It will induce sleep without any habit-forming medicine. This is good for tiny babies and elderly people. For adults, I would suggest fixing half of this and drinking the whole cup at bed time.   Mrs Clarence Miller & Mrs Susie Miller

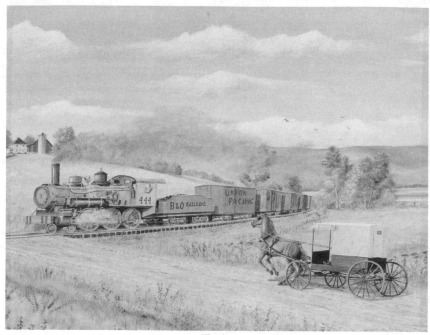

Train

To help calm your nerves, take 1 tsp. of celery seed in a cup of boiling water. Drink this as hot as you can, seeds and all.

A cup of chamomile tea is great for helping you relax. It's also a good remedy for the "baby blues". Chamomile tea is also safe enough to give to colicky or fussy babies.   Mrs Andy J Byler

Vitamin B-12 deficiency can produce serious nerve disorders, nerve disease of the arms and legs, a confused mental state, degeneration of the spinal cord and pernicious anemia, along with many other ailments.   Annie Petersheim

PARASITES
Garlic is good for getting rid of intestinal worms. Drink the garlic juice for best results.   Mrs Eli L Glick

To get rid of parasites, take at least 1 or 2 garlic and parsley capsules before going to bed. This can also help with colds. You could also use shell flour capsules for the parasites.   Lydia Swarey

2 T. water   1 tsp. caster oil
1 heaping tsp. sugar   1/2 tsp. turpentine
Take 8 - 9 drops of this in the morning, two mornings in a row. I've heard it's good to use this treatment every three months.

Put equal parts of fresh garlic, Extra Virgin Ariston, and olive oil and mix, put in a jar, set for 2 weeks. Dosage: little children 1 tsp. 3 evenings in a row, School age 1T., teenager 2T., and adults 3 T. Also 3 evenings in a row. This gets them in intestines. Repeat in 2 weeks.   Herman D Gingerich

POISON IVY/POISON OAK

To treat the affected area, rub the insides of a banana peel over it. To draw the poison out, put raw potato slices, cabbage or red beets on it.   Mrs Andy J Byler

To rid yourself of poison ivy, stir some alum into Vaseline. Put this mixture right on the affected area a few times or until it's gone.   Mrs Dan J Swartzentruber

For poison ivy, put olive oil on the affected area. This may sound simple, but my brother says it works like a charm the minute you put it on. He has an old doctor book from the 1800's, which is where he found this remedy.
                                                                    Mrs. John H Miller

For poison ivy itching, try washing the affected area with hot water, as hot as you can stand. Soda or vinegar can be added to the hot water.

Hold the affected area under hot water. The water should be as hot as the patient can stand. Hold the area under the hot water until the itching goes away. This remedy should provide about 8 hours of relief. The rash will still last for a week or two, but the itching is lessened which lessens the risk of infection.
                                                                Henry & Anna Schwartz

This is a home remedy that I received from a medical doctor, which proved very effective. Mix yellow sulfur with lard until you reach a paste consistency. Bathe the affected area and apply the sulfur paste over the entire area. Do this at least once a day for 3 days. The sulfur used to be available at drug stores, but you'd probably have to try a feed store now. For prevention, make sure that you wash the area that has come into contact with the poisonous plant with warm soapy water immediately.   M. Schwartz

Here's a remedy that works for poison ivy plus other sores or bruises. Take 1 qt. of burdock and plantain leaves. Mash them or chop them very fine in a heavy pan over low heat. Stir and chop until there is moisture. You may have to add a couple drops of water. Put moist pulp between two thin cloths over the area to be treated. The burdock is to draw out the swelling and the plantain (or pig ears) cures the ivy.

Soak the affected area in wood ashes for relief. This is also a good remedy for cuts and hard bruises.   Mrs Alvin Yoder

Try sponging ReaLemon juice over the affected area. This will soothe and halt the rash.

To relieve the itch of poison ivy, mix vinegar with an equal measure of water. Dab this frequently onto affected areas.   Mrs Mattie Ann Miller

Bathe the affected areas in sassafras tea. This should kill it after several applications. Another remedy is to heat whey or sour milk and pat it on with a cloth or cotton ball when it starts to itch. Always heat it first though.   Ida C Miller

Take ripe poke berries and rub the juice all over the affected area. Sprinkle cornstarch to the area to take away the stickiness of the poke juice. You may also put about 1 capful of chlorine bleach in the bath water. The cornstarch and poke juice mixture may be washed off with the bleach water, which will help to dry the affected area.   Annie J Peachey

Use jewelweed for relief of poison ivy.   Lucy Hackman

Rub rhubarb leaves on poison till it forms juice.   Simon S Schwartz

PROUD FLESH
Proud flesh is the tough, hard area around the nail bed of either the fingernails or toenails. To get rid of this, put alum on the affected area.   Mrs Andy J Byler

To cure proud or wild flesh, put some powdered alum on the affected area a few times a day.   Mrs Noah J Swartzentruber

Bandage powdered alum on to the red flesh overnight. In the morning the flesh will be brown and ready to crumble. You may need to do this more than once.
                                        Mrs Savilla Gingerich

Try putting some powdered alum on the proud flesh and then wrap the affected area with a bandage. In the morning you see it has turned brown.
                                        Elva Gingerich

RHEUMATISM
| 6 lemons | 6 oranges | 6 grapefruits |

Grind up peelings and all. Put 4 tablespoons Epsom Salts over this, next pour 1 quart boiling water over this and let stand overnight. Next morning put in a cloth bag and press out all the juice. Give a tablespoon of this juice 3 times a day. This is supposed to cure Rheumatism in 6 weeks time. Jerome took 3 tablespoons 3 times a day. Pain gone after 2 months.   Mrs Jerome Hochstetler

2 oz. tincture of black cohosh	1/2 oz. tincture of capsicum
2 oz. tincture of lobelia	2 oz. fluid extract mullein
1 oz. tincture prickly ash	1 pt. alcohol

A good liniment for Rheumatic, especially where joints are swollen.
                                        John J Miller

RINGWORM
I used to get ringworm occasionally. So whenever I saw he first sign of it, I would rub a little apple cider vinegar on the spot. It would sting, but soon the "thing" would go away. Even if I left one get a head start so that you could see the ring, it still worked.   William B Kilmer

Ringworm infestations will disappear when golden seal tea is regularly sipped at bedtime. Using the leaves of the plantain to make a tea, which should be sipped at bedtime, will quickly eliminate parasites also.   Henry & Anna Schwartz

Rub pine tar directly on the ringworm. Usually one application is all that is needed. This works well for man and beast.   Samuel J Bontrager

Put castor oil on the area 2 or 3 times a day.   Mrs. Levi S Miller

Vinegar is good to apply on ringworm.   Alvin Yoder

Use tea tree oil or peroxide on ring worm several times a day.
      William Beachy

SCABIES
Mix a small amount of sulfur with lard and put on the affected area twice a day (or more) until the scabies are gone. This has worked for me where doctor's medicine failed.   Joseph W Bontreger

SHINGLES
For shingles, apply vinegar or honey 4 times daily to the affected area.
      Mrs. Susie Miller

To ease the pain of shingles, gently pat on full strength vinegar. Do this at least four times a day and three times during the night. The discomfort will be much relieved.   Rebecca Miller

SKIN CARE
Pimples are evidence the body is trying to cleanse itself of toxins. Try fasting periodically as this will detoxify the body. Dab pimples with Listerine mouthwash and watch them disappear or use a mix of the juice of 2 garlic cloves with an equal amount of apple cider vinegar. (See also Body Cleanse)

Because sassafras tea purifies the blood, it could be taken for acne as well. Increase the effectiveness by also applying a compress soaked in warm tea to the affected area. Repeat this several times a day.   Henry & Anna Schwartz

For acne, take black currant seed oil or evening primrose oil capsules. A good dose would be 500 mg. 3 times a day. Do this for 3 months or until the acne clears up.
      Dan A Wengerd

For very sore skin or infected areas, use some wheat flour and warm water to make a paste. Add a little yeast and let it sit a little. Add some warm wood ash to thicken it. Put this on a piece of cloth and place the cloth on the wound. It may pull too hard if you leave it on too long.   Dan S Swartzentruber

For a body powder, mix 1/2 Baking Soda, 1/2 cornstarch, 1/2 baby powder or of your preference. Use daily.   Mary Detweiler

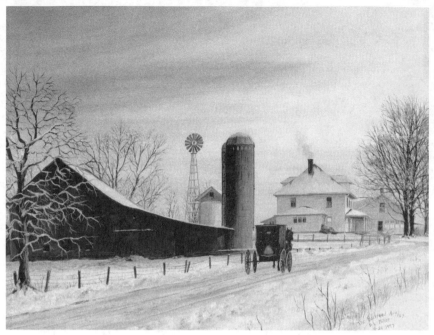

Winter Evening

Senica Lotion is good to soften and moisten roughed, chapped skin. It's also good for sore muscles'& joints, open sores and rashes. Just put it on and rub in.

Amos A Miller

Take the outside shell of walnuts and make a strong tea. Bathe all of the affected areas thoroughly.

Mrs J A Hershberger

For cracks around your fingernails and tips, use clear fingernail polish or Crazy glue right on the crack.

Calvin T Lambright

For pimples I had good results using Beta-Carotene 25,000 IU. (Provitamin A).

Amos Miller

Castor oil is good to get rid of moles and etc. Just rub a little on every day till gone. Also pulls pain. We warmed a cloth and put oil on. Put wherever pain is, then put plastic on top as you don't want oil on clothes. Leave on for the night. Throw away the rags if they get soiled too bad. This worked real well to pull the pain when my mother had cancer. But then she got so sick from the oil because she didn't have a gall bladder.

Wilmer E Schrock

Mix equal parts of glycerin, lemon juice, and white vinegar to use as a hand conditioner for dry skin problems, especially when working with concrete.

William Beachy

For soft, glowing skin, beat an egg white until nice and frothy and then add a tablespoon each of sweet clover honey and vinegar. Apply to the face and neck. Let dry completely, then sponge off with cool water.   Rebecca Miller

Work one tablespoon olive oil into one cup of thoroughly mashed, freshly picked, strawberries. Add 1/4 cup sweet clover honey. Use to revitalize the skin before bathing.   Rebecca Miller

SMOKING
Stop nicotine cravings by taking alka-seltzer. This will halt the withdrawal symptoms. (See also Body Cleanse)

SNAKE BITE
For snake bites, as soon as possible, slice an onion and hold a slice tight to the bite, if it turns green in 10 or 15 minutes turn the slice around. If it seems dry, cut it lightly or dampen it, than as that turns green put on a new slice. Keep it juicy. Also good for spider or hornet bites. One night after dark I got a snake bite. It started swelling before I got to the house. We kept onions on it all night. The next day I was able to go away. My dad believed in eating lots of onions to prevent gallstones or kidney stones and never had to operate on any.
David S & Polly Borntrager

SORE THROAT
For soothing a sore throat, warm some tomato juice and add a little red pepper, honey, salt, and whatever else you like. Gargle and sip this throughout the day. Very effective. Eating red beets will soothe a sore throat.   DeVon Miller

Take equal parts of honey, apple cider vinegar and lemon and gargle or sip often.

Gargle with vinegar, either straight or diluted with water. Add some salt for extra relief. The ratio for the ingredients is 1 T. vinegar, 1 T. water and 1/8 tsp. salt. Gargle every half hour and swallow a little each time.
Milton & Lizzie J Yoder; Mrs Clarence Miller

Different doctors have told us to put 1 tsp. salt in a glass with warm water and gargle 4 or more times daily until sore throat is gone.
Joseph W Bontreger; David & Treva Lambright; Daniel L Miller

Gargle with barberry tea to get relief from sore throat due to sinus drainage. This tea is also good for lungs, bowels or female disorders.   Amanda A. Miller

To relieve the pain of a sore throat caused by a cold, mix together 1/4 cup honey and 1/4 cup apple cider vinegar, take one tablespoon every four hours. May be taken more often if needed.   Sylvia L Shetler

For sore throats, make a solution of 1 pint warm water and 1 tsp. baking soda and 1 tsp. salt. Dissolve all the ingredients together and gargle 2 - 3 times per day.
Gingerich

For sore throat we use dried persimmon bark and make a strong tea. Gargle often, but if a child can't it is alright to swallow it.   Elmer Yoder

I woke up one morning at 4:00. My throat hurt so bad I couldn't swallow. I mixed equal parts of vinegar and honey and warmed it, sprayed my throat, went back to bed, and when I got up at 6:00 I didn't feel a sore throat.   Mary Detweiler

Sinus drainage can be greatly reduced by drinking 1 tsp. of vinegar mixed into a glass of water. This can also relieve dizziness.   Mattie Ann Miller

Make some sage tea to gain relief from a sore throat. You can also take a lemon and dip it in a little sugar and eat it straight.   Mrs J A Hershberger

For sore throat mix 1/2 T. ginger and 1 cup water. Gargle 3 times daily. We had very good results with this.   Gideon E Gingerich

SPLINTERS
Do you have a sliver that is almost impossible to get out? Finely grate some raw carrots and put them on the affected area until the sliver is out. This also works very well on drawing the soreness out of puncture wounds or similar sores. Red beets also work, but they stain more.   David W Brenneman

When you have a splinter in a hard to get to place, soak it several times a day with a handful of wood ashes in as warm water as you can stand. After a while the splinter is usually ready to pop out as it'll be slippery with the pus that has formed and is usually quite painless by then because wood ash works as a pain reliever also.   Mrs. Alvin Yoder

SPRAINS
Wrap the sprain with a home-cured bacon rind. If there are none available, scrape off the fat from some bacon with a knife and apply it to the area. Cover the sprain with a cloth.   William Miller

Keep a cold pack of 1 part rubbing alcohol and 2 parts water in a ziplock bag in freezer to place on sprains etc.   William Beachy

STOMACH UPSET
To ease an upset stomach, make a slice of toast and spread with butter. Crumble the buttered toast into hot milk and eat slowly.   Andy J. Byler

For an upset stomach when traveling, sip ginger tea before starting out. This really works! For a burning, acid stomach, stir into 1 cup of water 2 tsp. of baking soda and 1 tsp. sugar. Add 6 drops of oil of peppermint. Sip this slowly and you'll feel better quickly. Sip some Comfrey tea when you're not feeling quite up to par. Several cups can prevent many illnesses from getting you down. If suffering from colic and stomach spasms, try getting relief by drinking some chamomile tea. This tea can be given by spoonfuls to infants.   Henry & Anna Schwartz

To relieve that dull stomach ache, try taking Aloe Vera juice or gel and garlic/Echinacea extract.

Dissolve 1/2 teaspoon dry ginger in a half glass of warm water, or take two ginger capsules with warm water.

When your stomach is feeling upset, heat some milk and pour it over toast, then eat it slowly. Another remedy is to take 1 tsp. of apple cider vinegar in a glass of water and drink slowly.   Mrs. Andy J. Byler

For an upset stomach, mix some warm water and nutmeg and drink the mixture.   Perry J. Miller

Mix 1 qt. of water, 2 T. white sugar, and 1/2 tsp. salt. Mix well and drink. Another one is to eat potato mush and meat with gravy. This will help to settle the stomach.

For vomiting mix: 1 cup frozen orange concentrate, 8 tsp. ReaLemon juice, 4 tsp. Karo, Crushed ice to make 1 pint. Give 2 tsp. every 15 min. to settle stomach. This works amazingly well.   William Beachy

Take a T. vinegar twice a day for upset stomach and diarrhea.
                                                    Daniel A Hershberger

For upset stomach lick on salt till you are satisfied. I had very good results with this.   Gideon E Gingerich

STREP THROAT
Make a tea of 1/4 tsp. myrrh gum, 1/4 tsp. golden seal, and 1 tsp. of white oak bark. Gargle with this as often as possible. It's very bitter, but has amazing results.
                                                    Mrs. Andy Keim

STUTTERING
Stuttering, especially in children, seems to be helped by a vitamin B supplement. About 10 mg of B1 should be taken per day. It is recommended to take a B complex supplement.   Mrs. Alvin Yoder

SUNBURNS
For relief from sunburns, apply some Aloe Vera from the plant, full strength onto the affected area. This also applies to flash burns from a welder. If the eyes become burned, squeeze the juice from the plant into the eye. Put two drops in each eye. This is a good remedy for all kinds of burns.

For sunburn relief use apple cider vinegar on the sunburned area.

SWELLING
If the body is beset with toxins in the system, and there is swelling in the legs, try drinking some dandelion leaf tea. This will help to cleanse the system of toxins. Another good remedy for swelling in the legs and feet is to sip on a tea made with alfalfa.   Henry & Anna Schwartz

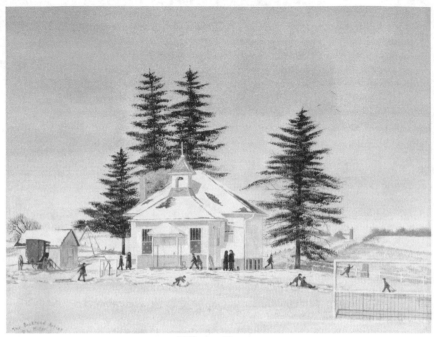

Winter Recess

TICK BITES

If tick bites get sore, tie a charcoal salve on them. Make the salve out of a few tsp. of charcoal and enough water so that it stays on a thin cloth, but still soaks well. Change the cloth when it becomes dry. Make sure that you do not use the charcoal again because once it has been used on a sore, it becomes full of toxins.

Emanuel Yoder Family

Mom discovered a mole on her back (she couldn't see it), so several days later she got Dad to look at it. To their horror, it was a tiny tick, that stuck hard. Then mom admitted to not feeling very good that day. The next morning mom told us about it. We picked plantain leaves in the lawn, rubbed the leaves to crush them until they got juicy. (Preferably the leaf still hangs together.) And put it on the bite. Changing it at least 2 times daily for 1 week. She also drank activated charcoal according to the directions for snake bite. 2 Tbsp. every 2 hours for 3 doses. Then 1 tsp. every 4 hours for 24 hours. Each dose followed by 2 glasses of water. Mom then took a teaspoonful every evening for several days. The charcoal is like a dust and can easiest be mixed with water (for drinking) by putting some water in a pint jar, adding the charcoal, turning on the lid and shaking. Drink it with a straw if you want to.

Mary E Beachy

I had a pediatrician tell me what she believes is the best way to remove a tick. This is great, because it works in those places where it's sometimes difficult to get to with tweezers: between toes, in the middle of a head full of dark hair, etc. Apply a glob of liquid soap to a cotton ball. Cover the tick with the soap-soaked cotton ball and let it stay on the repulsive insect for a few seconds (15-20), after

74

which the tick will come out on its own and be stuck to the cotton ball when you lift it away. This technique has worked every time I've used it (frequently), and it's much less traumatic for the patient and easier for me. Unless someone is allergic to soap, I can't see that this would be damaging in any way. I even had my doctor's wife call me for advice because she had one stuck to her back and she couldn't reach it with tweezers. She used this method and immediately called me back to say, 'It worked!'

TOOTH CARE
To relieve a toothache, wet a small piece of cotton with vanilla and put it on the aching tooth.   Enos R. Byler

Chew on whole garlic cloves to relieve tooth pain. I've gotten good results from this.   Ida C Miller

For toothache relief, take a Comfrey leaf and chew it with the tooth that hurts.
                                                                                  Jacob Christner

To rid yourself of a nasty toothache, put some pure Epsom Salts directly on the sore tooth. This will last about six months before you suffer from another toothache.
                                                                                  Gingerich

To take the pain away from a cavity, take a whole clove and place it in the cavity. Bite down hard and hold it there. Clove oil will also work. Mrs Andy J Byler

Here's an idea to inspire your children to keep their teeth clean. Set a timer at 3 minutes in the bathroom and tell them to brush until it goes off.
                                                                                  Noah J Petersheim

To ensure white teeth and sweet breath, brush with this special mixture.
1 T. baking soda   1 T. salt   1 tsp. lemon juice
1 drop of peppermint oil   Henry & Anna Schwartz

When mom got her teeth pulled she used cream of tartar for pain.
                                                                                  William B Kilmer

Olive oil is good for toothache. Take a cotton swab or Q-tip and rub on aching tooth.   Wilmer E Schrock

If your teeth seem yellow or discolored, always use peroxide before brushing and brush twice a day.   Raymond Schwartz

Split a raisin in half and put black pepper in between and put on the tooth that hurts.   Amos Miller

ULCERS
For ulcers drink plenty of eggnog. (See also Body Cleanse) Mrs Andy J Byler

VARICOSE VEINS

To relieve problems with varicose veins, take Butcher's Broom. Vetebrae out of place in your lower back will inhibit blood circulation.

You can heal varicose veins in one month. Pat some full-strength vinegar onto the offending veins twice a day. Each morning and evening, drink a glass of water with two tsp. of vinegar in it.   Henry & Anna Schwartz

WARTS

To get rid of warts, put warm castor oil on some gauze and apply this to the wart 3 times a day for half an hour each time. Within 3 weeks the warts should disappear.   Lydia Petersheim

Here's a remedy to rid yourself of warts. Put tea tree oil on the wart both morning and evening. They will soon disappear.   Milton & Lizzie J Yoder

Drop a little pure apple cider vinegar on the wart and cover it immediately with baking soda. Put on as much baking soda as you can pile on and leave it there ten minutes. Repeat this procedure three times a day and in three or four days the wart will be gone. This is a good remedy for corns.   Ada Swartzentruber

Tie a piece of garlic on the wart, changing it twice a day. Garlic should be cut in small pieces so a wet surface contacts the wart. Sometimes this takes a week or two. If the wart is stubborn, pull it out, roots and all, then apply the garlic treatment. It heals up nicely with hardly a scar.   Samuel J Bontrager

Mix red pepper with vinegar to make a paste. Apply this on the warts and put a Band-Aid on. Leave on for 2 days and 2 nights. This at times is very painful. Be sure not to get it on skin, because it's too strong. Just put on the wart. Take the Band-Aid off at the end of 2 days and nights, even if the warts are not gone. Some don't find out when they disappear. Don't get your hands wet at the time the Band-Aid is on.   Fannie Schrock

WHOOPING COUGH

Take 3 or 4 chestnut leaves to 1 pint boiling water. Steep to a tea and sweeten (honey is good). Let the children drink this 5 to 6 times a day.
                    Mrs Atlee N Troyer

Make a tea by boiling 1 tsp. of wild cherry bark and 1 T. red sage in a pint of water. Take 1 tsp. of this five times a day.   Mary S Yoder

Simmer 1 pt. water, 1 cup flaxseed, and 1 thinly sliced lemon slowly for 4 hours. Don't bring it to a boil. Strain it while the liquid is still hot and add enough water to make 1 pt. If it's less than a pint add 2 oz. honey. For an adult dose use 1 T. four times a day, plus 1 T. after each coughing spell. For children use 1 tsp. four times a day, plus 1 tsp. after each coughing spell.   Mrs Levi S Miller

WOUNDS

One of the oldest remedies was to apply honey to the wound. Bacteria disappears quickly according to several studies conducted by several doctors. Even wounds

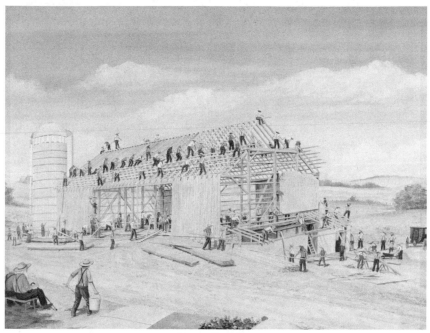

Barn Raising

refusing to heal with antibiotics, had completely healed in one week. Twelve surgery patients had honey applied to their incisions and were completely healed up in 3-8 weeks. Weary German soldiers on the battlefield in World War I used honey on their wounds to heal quickly.

Use lobelia for bumps and bruises on both children and adult's heads. I like to keep it on hand for when someone has a fall. It is really soothing and helps relieve pain very quickly. It also helps the swelling to go down.

Whole wheat flour mixed with the yolk of one egg, along with some honey and turpentine will draw, cleanse and heal any sore or ulcer. Mrs John Detweiler

For injuries with painful black and blue bumps, wet a rag with vinegar and hold it on the bruise and the pain will soon leave. A bump will be less, do not use on open cuts.   David J Wickey

Crushed cranberries make a good poultice for wounds, such as dog or cat bites.
Atlee E Miller

For a puncture wound such as caused by stepping on a nail, soak in peroxide and epsom salts. Soak a washcloth with pure apple cider vinegar, place it on the wound, cover it with a plastic bag and pull on a large sock to keep it in place overnight. Repeat until healed. Amazing! No more hot, feverish or swollen. Delilah Stoll

Cut a lemon in half and place the cut side on the open sore overnight. Put castor oil packs onto the wound and let them soak.   Joseph W Schrock

To keep from getting infections in puncture wounds, cuts, etc. take several burdock and mullein leaves and soak in boiling water for several minutes. Put wet leaves on the sore. If the leaves get dry, wet them again in same tea. Wrap the wet leaves around the wound for extra help. This is a good remedy to draw out infection and soreness from any wounds. You can even hold the affected area right in the tea if possible. Charcoal water is also very good to soak sores in to take the infection away and keep infection from setting in. Use 1 T. charcoal powder in 1 qt. warm water. Soak as often as needed to keep redness down.   Emanuel Yoder Family

Green or dried burdock leaves are really good for healing wounds and taking soreness out of strained muscles and broken bones. To use, soak the leaves in hot water just a few seconds. Don't soak them long enough to color the water, just enough to soften the leaves and then put them on the affected area.
                                        Abie J Stutzman

Put some vinegar in hot water to draw out pain and infection from cuts, etc. It will also draw out slivers so they could easily be removed. For long or deep cuts, put a band aid crosswise over the wound and draw together very tightly. This can prevent the need for stitches in some cuts.   Mrs Jacob L Miller

Plantain leaves picked fresh from your yard and rolled into a poultice consistency have great drawing power. They can be put on splinters, bug bites, etc.
                                        Mrs Andy Keim

For puncture wounds or open cuts that are painful, pour boiling water over wood ashes and let cool to the warmth you can put your hand into. Now soak the sore area in it for 30-60 minutes. It will draw out any infection. Use approximately several handfuls of ash to a gallon of water. You can tell when you've got enough ashes in the water when the affected area can feel the tingle or bite. Use just enough to make it tingle and use as hot water as one can stand. The water will look "unfit" but this does wonders. Sometimes soaking only once was enough, but if the area was more painful, it took more soakings. This remedy never fails to draw the soreness out and speed the healing. The wound will come out looking nice and clean.   Lena Yoder; Milton & Lizzie J Yoder; Mrs Toby H Yoder; William Miller; M Schwartz

Take 3/4 cup of milk of magnesia and 1 tsp. of sugar and mix well. Put this on an open sore. A nurse told me she hasn't seen the sore yet that this mixture hasn't healed.   Mrs John Detweiler

A good remedy for sores of any kind, even if they're infected, is to take a small red beet and shave it into small pieces. Make a poultice with it and put it on the wound. This will draw out pain and infection. Another remedy is to soak bread in milk and put it on the sore area. Make sure to fasten it so that it stays in place. Use this at bedtime and in the morning you should see some improvement. Repeat this if necessary.   Sam E Miller

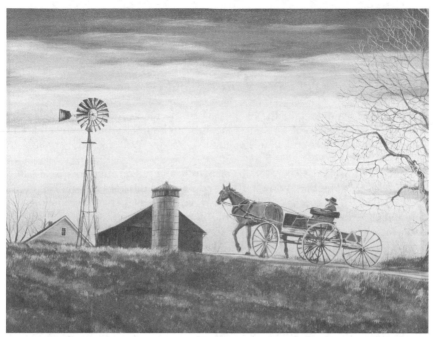

Sunset

When there is persistent bleeding, wash the wound off with pure cider vinegar. The vinegar causes the blood to coagulate.   Mrs Harley Miller

Soak the wound or put in strong Comfrey tea twice a day. This is also good to draw out pain and for staph infections. Also tie burdock leaves on the bad cuts or infections.

To fight infection in a puncture wound, soak the wound in Epsom Salts for 10-15 minutes. Put some Union Salve on a bandage to dress the wound. You can also use plantain leaves that grow in the yard and add some Aloe Vera to dress the wound.   Enos R Byler

For deep cuts that had o be stitched our family doctor said to wash it off a couple times a day with warm water and Dawn dishwashing soap. Keep the cut clean and dry with no salve. For scrapes, nail punctures, etc. soak affected area in approximately 1 gallon of water with a dash of Dreft Soap.   William Beachy

Wipe the blood off and put peppermint oil directly on the wound, then bandage it. If you wash the cut, the peppermint oil should be applied before any water. This is our number one remedy. Another option is if the cut should become infected put honey on it and bandage it with tape or a Band-Aid. If you need to stop the bleeding of a wound, put cayenne pepper directly on the cut. It can be powdered or a tincture.   Samuel J Bontrager

For deep cuts that need sutures, mix cayenne pepper and golden seal in a Vaseline base. Fill the cut and pull together with a butterfly bandage. Red pepper kills infection and golden seal pulls together skin much better than sutures. This will leave no ridges and usually no scars.   Mrs Andy Keim

Disinfect wounds with Tea Tree oil first.

For puncture wounds, take the heel of a loaf of bread (preferably homemade) and soak it in heated milk. Drain it some and put it on the wound while it is still warm. Wrap the bread and all in a bandage.   Mrs. Walter (Clara) Troyer

For stubborn infection, soak bread in warm milk and put on affected area at night. Wrap a cloth around that. Wrap a plastic bag around the poultice and keep it on overnight. I used this in the evening before going to bed and by the next morning, you could see the infection was a lot better. Sometimes this draws out all the infection over night. This has taken care of infection for our son after we had him to the doctor and the doctor's medicine failed.   Joseph W Bontreger

I keep a red wash cloth in a easy to find place to wash cuts and scratches that bleed. The children do not see the blood on the red cloth. Tears are soon gone and they're ready to return to play!!   Joe E T Schwartz

We put a can sprayer on our peroxide bottle to spray into wounds. It works very nice and not so much goes to waste   Joe E T Schwartz

Using masking tape for use with gauze for wounds and cuts works much better then tape from Pharmacies etc. It sticks better.   Joe E T Schwartz

YEAST INFECTION
Used 4 tsp. vinegar to a pint of water for a douche. Acidophilus is also good for yeast infection, take 4 every 4 hours.   Amos Miller

For relief from yeast infections, get a vitamin called Acidophilus. You should be able to locate this at most health food stores. Another nutrient to take is zinc. The daily recommended dosage is 15 mg. Taking too much zinc, though, is not recommended as it could cause a copper deficiency. Another good remedy is yogurt. Feeding your children yogurt is an easy way to help with the yeast infection.

WEIGHT LOSS

WEIGHT LOSS SMORGASBORD

It is estimated that 61% of Americans are overweight and eat 3 times more than is really needed for robust health and vigor. Overweight people are the unlucky victims of a distorted body chemistry. We all know people who eat very little-- they literally starve themselves out of good health and are still overweight. We also know of people who can "eat like a horse" and are still very skinny. Why is it that some people can eat a big meal and still feel hungry? The issue is not in the amount of food we eat. The body chemistry of an overweight person is different from that of a naturally skinny person. When you understand this dif- ference and how to handle it, losing weight becomes much easier than you ever thought possible.

There are many things people can become addicted to: alcohol, nicotine, drugs, overeating, etc. An addiction of overeating is much harder to overcome than all the others put together. Contrary to popular opinion, overweight people usu- ally have more willpower than almost anyone else. Most overweight people have gone on near-starvation diets for lengths of time that others would not have endured. Your body doesn't need alcohol or nicotine. It is much easier to give them up completely than to consume them in small quantities. Our bodies can't do without food and it is this constant "teasing" of our body with calories that makes it difficult to whip the overeating addiction. Someone can literally be overwhelmed with thoughts of food.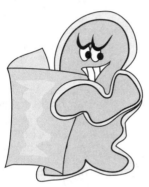

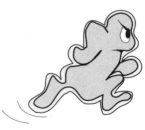 If you are like most overweight people, you have gone searching for the perfect diet. After a number of weeks of dieting, you just can't stand it anymore so you quit. With a vengeance, you are absolutely driven to eat and eat and eat to make up for all the suffering you went through. And like most people you will gain back everything you lost, plus some. So like most people you go looking for another diet which only produces the same result. Calorie count- ing doesn't work either. It just gets harder as time passes. These kinds of diets don't work in the long run. Your willpower can't stand up to a day-in and day-out gnawing hunger. Even if you could withstand this constant torture, what good would it do if you are always miserable and hungry? Is there anything that can be done for a runaway hunger . . . a plan that will break up the hunger cycle so you can think about something else besides food . . . a plan that lets you get a little fun out of life . . . a plan that can let you eat cake once in awhile and lose weight too? There is in fact an easy answer to all of these problems described so far.

Metabolism is the life force which regulates our body tem- perature, controls the healing of cuts and wounds, turns food into energy, controls secretions of our body's fluids and hormones, and performs other important body functions. For most people, metabolism loses its efficiency with age, about 1% per year after 25.

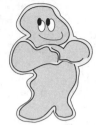

It is a low blood sugar level that tells us we are hungry. Now what happens when we eat something? Our blood sugar level goes up. Our body produces insulin to take out any excess sugar in our bloodstream and stores it in our liver for later use. At least that is how it is supposed to work. This is also where the problem comes in. Unfortunately, if you are overweight, your body has a tendency to produce too much insulin too fast which takes out most of the sugar in your bloodstream and you are right back to being hungry again. So now you know the secret of why overweight people are overweight. They are hungry almost all the time! And it's not their fault! So if we can improve our metabolism we can whip the hunger lion that wants to overtake us.

It is very easy to raise your blood sugar level; eat something with sugar in it. There are two basic kinds of sugar. Fructose is the sugar contained in fruits. Sucrose is the sugar contained in candy, desserts and other processed foods. They basically raise your blood sugar level the same amount. Blood sugar level goes up fast if you eat something that is sweet. Have you ever heard of someone becoming overweight by eating fruits? No! So avoid eating <u>sucrose</u> sugars like the plague. When you get hungry, eat a slice of fruit, any fruit. Better yet, "eat before you eat." It takes about 20 minutes for your blood sugar level to rise high enough to not feel hungry. Eat a slice of fruit about 30 minutes before you sit down to eat. This will do exactly what your mother always said it will do. "Don't eat so close to dinner time. You won't be hungry anymore." And she was right.

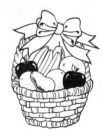

Eat breakfast. If you are overweight you probably skip breakfast, eat a light lunch and have a huge evening meal. Turn it completely around! Eat a good breakfast and lunch and a light evening meal. Eat your evening meal no later than 6 PM if possible with no bedtime snack. (Sumo wrestlers in Japan win by pushing their opponent out of a ring. They gorge themselves just before going to bed so they will gain weight.) Remember, keep it light and early.

Diet every other day. Sound too simple? It is important though! This dieting will last much longer than if you diet every day for a few weeks. One lady lost 40 lbs. by doing just this.

Drink at least 8 glasses of water a day. An added advantage is if it is cold water. This will cause your body to use more energy.

Take 2 teaspoons of real lemon juice after every meal.

82

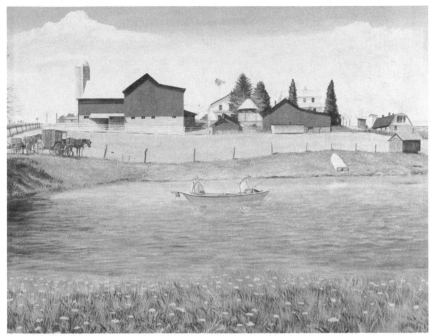

Fishing

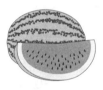 Do a watermelon flush. Eat all the watermelon you want during the day, nothing else. You will be astonished when you weigh yourself the next morning. Not only will you lose weight fast but this is a remarkable body cleanser. You will feel more calm and your mind will be clearer. It's very easy and it works!

Take 2 teaspoons of the below mixture every 2 hours during the day for a month. Mix together 1 cup finely shredded raw beets, the juice of 1/2 a raw lemon and 2 T. of olive oil.

 Another fast weight loss technique is to eat nothing but papayas or mangos for a day or so. These fruits have a laxative and a diuretic effect. Some people can lose more weight this way than being on a strict water-only fast.

Consume calcium daily whether in calcium rich foods or as a good supplement. It not only is an excellent pain killer but will make other nutrients in your food bioavailable to your body. It will keep your body fluids alkaline. If body fluids are acidic, disease and illness will be rampant.

Apple cider vinegar will supply you with many of the nutrients of which you are deficient. Many people are deficient of the minerals found in apple cider vinegar. This will make up for deficient nutrients your body might be "hungry" for.

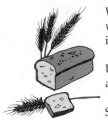

Wheat germ. Add this ingredient to your diet such as eating whole wheat bread or adding wheat germ to your cereal. It is rich in the B vitamins.

Use Brewer's yeast in your foods. It is chock full of B vitamins and will make you feel much better.

Sweat everyday. Your skin eliminates more than 60% of our body toxins. Your health and skin quality will improve dramatically. Have plain ol' fashioned fun. Your enthusiasm or the lack of it will effect your health. Many overweight people are bored and they turn to eating as a release from their pit. This is not an afterthought. This is important! For every pound of "overweightness" you lose, you must add a pound of excitement to your life.

Now, the best thing! This will be your most powerful health and beauty secret. If you do the following on a regular basis your skin will clear up and soften. Your eyes will sparkle again. Your hair will glisten. Your eyesight will improve. You will have a fresh, clean-scrubbed appearance about you. The food we eat has many impurities in it. If our metabolism is distorted, these impurities are not purged and burned off from our system. These toxins lodge in the cells of our body and create the ideal environment for all kinds of disease and sickness. Now here is what you do. Do a short, periodic fast. Too simple? Some people have the mentality that to accomplish something big such as to lose weight, it must be hard and complicated. Sometimes the most simple things 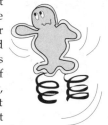 work the best. Some people fast in the extreme by only drinking water. Others use fresh juices from fruits or vegetables. Still others fast by eating only 6 crackers and the water or juice. Some like to fast every Monday or twice a week. However you do it will give your metabolism a chance to burn off the impurities and eliminate toxins which have accumulated. Your metabolism will stabilize. Your tongue will become coated and you will have foul breath. These are signs that it's working!

You should never go on a long fast without medical advice. But these short, periodic fasts are very beneficial. In the Bible, the story is given of two men who went up to the temple to pray. The one was a Pharisee and one of his good works he reminded God about was that he fasted twice a week. His self-righteous attitude stank pretty bad but somehow they had figured out how they could fast for obtaining optimum health. Fasting is considered one of the easiest ways to lose weight. Just drink a lot of water!

(See also Body Cleanse I)

To control the overly active appetite, try drinking several cups of red clover tea each day. To take some inches off the waistline, try drinking a glass of water with 2 tsp. of vinegar in it at each meal. This will take an inch from your waist in 2 months.

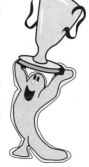

Henry & Anna Schwartz

To control the appetite, begin each meal with a nice bowl of freshly picked lettuce, dressed with two tablespoons of vinegar.   Atlee E Miller

Old-timers felt honey was nature's way to easy weight loss. Mix two teaspoons of honey into a glass of water and drink it 1/2 hour before each meal. You will melt away excess pounds.   Rebecca Miller

Drink a glass of water with 1 T. apple cider vinegar 15-30 minutes before each meal to lose weight and helps with fibromyalgia and joint pain.
                    Johnny Miller

Apple cider vinegar is helpful in melting away excess pounds. Simply drink a glass of warm water, with a single teaspoon of apple cider vinegar stirred in, before each meal, it moderates the over robust appetite and melts away fat.
                    Sylvia L Shetler

MIRACLE TEA
2 tsp honey   2 tsp apple cider vinegar
Mix into a glass of regular tea. Sipping just 2 teaspoons of miracle tea at each meal can produce a weight loss of up to 10 pounds a month.   Dr Jarvis

Eat raw whole foods as much as possible.

SALVES

ASTHMA COUGH SALVE
4 oz. Vaseline   1/2 oz. camphor gum   1/2 oz. menthol crystals
Melt the Vaseline in a small stainless steel pan. Shave the camphor and add the menthol crystals. Heat on low heat until melted. Pour in small jars. When you need to use this, exhale all that you can, then inhale as deep as possible. Hold your breath and exhale through your mouth. This is very good for a cough. Put a little of this in the hollow of your throat and rub in really well. This is also good for small children.

COMFREY SALVE
This works for burns, abrasions, diaper rash, chapped hands, cuts, etc. Harvest about a grocery bag of clean comfrey. With scissors, cut into narrow strips and fill a large pot. Add just enough water to cover comfrey - packing it down well. Simmer on low heat all day, stirring occasionally. Cool overnight and strain off liquid. Add 1 1/2 quarts olive oil or cooking oil to comfrey tea and replace on stove, on medium heat at first to evaporate all the water. This process will take 6-8 hours and must be watched carefully; as you get less water, turn down the heat. Stir more frequently toward the end and don't allow to burn. You will see the fine particles of comfrey clumping together at the bottom, and the bubbling will decrease as you get close to complete evaporation. Add 1-2 ounces of tea tree oil (melaleuca) if you have it. It is a wonderful antiseptic and antifungal. Add 1/2 pound beeswax to thicken the salve, and pour into jelly jars, or any small jar that you can get your fingers into. As it cools it will harden.
                                                    Deborah Moore -Midwife

DRAWING SALVE
For a good drawing salve, take some lard and add flour until you reach the right consistency.   Atlee Miller Family

HEALING SALVE
1 lb. lard   1/2" cube of beeswax
4 tsp. oil of spike   1 tsp. rosin
Melt lard and add wax. Bring to almost boiling then add the rosin. Take outside and add oil of spike (because it smells bad) and cool.

HOMEMADE SALVE
1 lb. resin   1 lb. beeswax
1 pint linseed oil   1 lb. fresh lard
Mix all ingredients together and put on the back of your stove. Simmer for three hours, stirring often. This is a very effective salve for any wound.
                                                  Menno & Malinda Miller

Pick fresh Plantain leaves, fill a clean jar, fill jar a second time with olive oil, dislodging any air bubbles, covering all the plant material. Label jar with date and let set out of direct sunlight for 6 weeks. Make sure jar is placed on a surface that will not be marred by the oil. The oil will go through several stages and fun to watch. But will ooze a little. After 6 weeks pour off the oil and squeeze out plant material.   Wilmer E Schrock

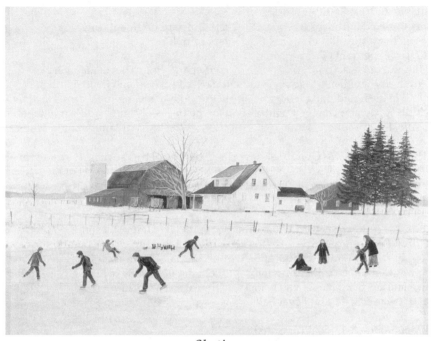

Skating

To every oz. of oil, add 1 T grated beeswax and content of Vitamin E capsule to preserve the salve. Heat oil stirring constantly, till wax is melted, less then a minute. We've had just as good luck with the salve as the leaves.

Wilmer E Schrock

To a pint of hot Apple Cider Vinegar, add 2 tablespoons of Powdered Cayenne (Capsicum) and 1 tablespoon of Golden seal Root. Cover and boil gently for 10 minutes. Cool then add a qt of Rubbing Alcohol and 2 oz. of Gum Myrrh. Keep this covered and let stand 5 or 6 days shaking well every day. Makes a wonderful natural liniment. This liniment will sting somewhat and heat up the skin. Unlike other liniments, it's not injurious to the skin, but rather provides a marvelous stimulating effect. Use freely as needed.   Fannie Schrock

INFLAMMATION SALVE
Take a gallon of unsalted lard, one large handful of rue, and 7 to 9 eggs. Put the lard in a kettle big enough so it can boil up. Heat the lard and put it in the rue and let simmer for at least 15 minutes. Then beat the eggs and put that on top of the rue, and let simmer awhile longer. Then turn the rue and eggs over. When the lard gets a brown color like brown lard, it should be done. Throw the eggs and rue out and strain the rest of the mixture. Stir it while it's cooling. This is a very good healing salve for sores, boils, etc.   Jonas A. Weaver

LUNG FEVER SALVE

1 c. unsalted lard
2 tsp. turpentine liquid
1 tsp. peppermint oil
Handful of black root

2 tsp. mustard ointment (salve)
1 tsp. camphor
2 T. salt
1 c vinegar   (ingredients may vary)

Put these ingredients together and melt it over heat. I spread it on a cloth or dip a cloth in the liquid. Ring it out and apply the cloth while it's still warm. Have two cloths ready and change them as soon as the one cools off or add a a hot water bottle. Do this for one hour.   William P Emma Miller

This (the above) was Grandma's favorite in her bag of tricks! Yuck! I can still smell it. She used it on me so often, just a whiff of it brings back a bushel of memories! But she says it's a sure cure for chest colds. Just make sure you have some on hand always!   Linda (Willis) Bontrager

3 oz. rosin, 3 oz. beeswax, 2 oz. camphor (pulverized, it comes in 1 oz. blocks.), 2 drams oil of turpentine, 2 drams oil of cedar, 1 lb. Lard. Melt lard and rosin on low heat, add camphor, and put cover on lightly so camphor won't evaporate. Stir now and then until camphor is all melted. Put the oils in just before you put in small jars or whatever you want it in when it's still warm enough to pour. Long ago it was called Lung Fever Salve.   Fannie Schrock

(Pneumonia, Asthma, Bronchitis)
In 1 1/2 qt. pan:
1 lemon sliced (washed well)   1 T. honey (or 2)   4 c. water
          Bring to a boil, then add:
2 tsp. thyme   2 tsp. plantain
Let steep 10-15 min. Strain. Pour into thermos. Keep hot. Sip 1/2 c. at a time. May use this recipe for whooping cough. Use same first part plus 1 c. flax seed. Simmer 4 hours. If there's less than 1 qt., add water to make 1 qt. Dose: 2 T. four times a day and after coughing spells. Use less for children.   Delilah Stoll

MARIGOLD COMPOUND SALVE

Gently heat 2 1/2 cup pure lard and 1 cup Vaseline. After it is melted and warm to the touch, add 2 heaping handfuls of marigold flowers and foliage, 1 handful Comfrey leaves and 1 handful of plantain leaves. Add 1 tsp. turmeric, also. Cover this with a tight fitting lid and let stand at room temperature for 24 hours. Reheat, strain and put in jars. This remedy is good for chapped lips and hands, diaper rash, cuts, bruises, etc.   Mrs Moses Z Stoltzfus

PNEUMONIA SALVE

6 oz. white rosin
4 oz. camphor gum
4 drams oil of turpentine

6 oz. bees wax
4 drams balsam Peru
4 drams oil of cider

Mix together in an old kettle with 12 oz. lard. Heat until all is melted, then strain into jars and cover, tightly. To use, spread the salve on a cloth, apply to the chest. Cover with a very warm flannel cloth.

WILD CHERRY COUGH SYRUP

Prepare wild cherries as for jelly: sort and clean, add enough water to cover berries and simmer 20-30 minutes. Mash the cherries and let cool enough to check taste after sweetening. Strain off juice. Add honey to sweeten. Reheat for canning process. Pour hot liquid into pint jars, process in hot water bath five minutes. If you have purple coneflower (Echinacea), add 1-2 clean leaves to each jar before filling with syrup.   Deborah Moore -Midwife

LINIMENT

This is a good remedy for sore muscles, sore throat, stiff joints, and phlebitis. Just rub the following ointment onto the surface of the affected area. Beat 6 egg whites until well beaten and add 4 oz. rectified turpentine. Beat in 1 oz. eucalyptus oil, 1/2 oz. olive oil and 2 oz. spirit of camphor. Next beat in 1 oz. sweet spirit of nitro, 1/2 oz. liquid capsicum, 1/4 oz. peppermint oil, 1 oz. wintergreen oil. Beat this all thoroughly and add 4 oz. Aloe Vera lotion and bottle the mixture.

For liniment mix 1 pint vinegar and 1/2 cup cayenne pepper boil together for 4 minutes. I had very good results with this.   Gideon E Gingerich

1/2 pt. good strong vinegar   1/2 pt. turpentine   1 egg
Shake well. This is a strong liniment!   Sammie & Kathryn Schrock

WHOOPING COUGH MEDICINE

Take one lemon and slice it thin. Add 1/2 pint of flax seed and one quart water. Simmer, but do not boil for four hours. Strain while hot and add two ounces of honey. If there is less than a pint of mixture, add water to make a pint. Dose: One tablespoon four times a day and, in addition, a dose after each severe fit of coughing. This remedy has never been known to fail. A cure being affected in four to five days if given before or when the child first whoops. Will help ease the coughing by allowing the phlegm to be passed out through the stool.

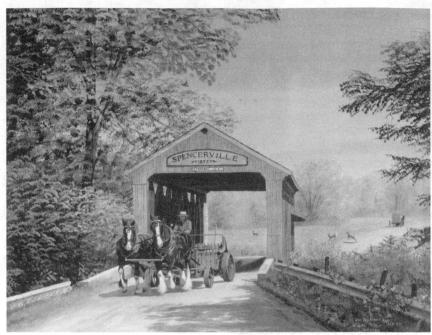

Ben & Alice

BASIC H, BASIC G, Etc.
Shaklee products are available from its distributors. Call
1-800-SHAKLEE (742-5533) to find one near you.

If you have a remedy the works, please send it to our address near the front of the book for our consideration.

INDEX

A

ALLERGIES 11
ANEMIA 11
ANTIOXIDANTS 11
ANXIETY 12
APPENDICITIS 12
ARTERIES 12
ARTHRITIS 13
ASTHMA 14
ASTHMA COUGH SALVE 86
ATHLETE'S FOOT 15

B

BABY COLDS 4
BABY WIPES 4
BEDWETTING 15
BED SORES 15
BLADDER INFECTIONS 61
BLEEDING 15
BLOOD POISONING 16
BODY CLEANSER 21
BODY CLEANSER I 17
BODY CLEANSER II 19
BRONCHITIS 21
BURNS 22

C

CANCER 23,24,26
CANKER SORES 26
CHICKEN POX 26
CHOLESTEROL 26
CLEAR THINKING 26
COLDS 27
COLON 21
COMFREY SALVE 86
CONSTIPATION 34
COOLING OFF 46
COUGH 27
COUGH SYRUP 89
CROUP 27

D

DEPRESSION 46
DIABETES SORES 44
DIARRHEA 46
DIURETIC TEA 44
DIZZINESS 44
DRAWING SALVE 86
DROPSY 44
DROWSINESS 45

E

EAR CARE 45
EDEMA 44
ESSIAC BLEND 24
EYE CARE 47

F

FERTILITY 47
FEVER 48
FLU 49
FLUID RETENTION 44
FOOD POISONING 50
FOOT CARE 50
FROSTBITE 50
FUSSY BABIES 9

G

GALL STONES 19,50

H

HAIR CARE 51
HEADACHE 51
HEAD LICE 52
HEALING SALVE 86
HEALTH MAINTENANCE 52
HEART ATTACKS 58
HEAT RASH 62
HEMORRHOIDS 62
HICCUPS 62
HIVES 63
HOMEMADE SALVE 86
HOT FLASHES 63

HOXSEY FORMULA 26

I

INDIGESTION 63
INFLAMMATION SALVE 87
INSECT STINGS 63
INSOMNIA 60
INTESTINAL DISTRESS 61
ITCHING 61

J

JAUNDICE 9,61

K

KIDNEY 61

L

LAXATIVE 63
LINIMENT 89
LIVER 19,21
LOW BLOOD SUGAR 63
LUNG FEVER SALVE 88

M

MARIGOLD COMPOUND SALVE 88
MEMORY 63
MENOPAUSE PROBLEMS 63
MENSTRUAL CRAMPS 64
MONO 64
MORNING SICKNESS 64
MOTION SICKNESS 64
MOUTHWASH 64
MUSCLE ACHES 64

N

NERVOUSNESS 65
NURSING MOTHERS 10

P

PARASITES 66

PNEUMONIA 27
PNEUMONIA SALVE 88
POISON IVY 67
POISON OAK 67
PROUD FLESH 68

R

RHEUMATISM 68
RINGWORM 68

S

SCABIES 69
SHINGLES 69
SINUS 27
SKIN CARE 69
SKIN RASHES 10
SMOKING 71
SNAKE BITE 71
SORE EYES 10
SORE THROAT 71
SPLINTERS 72
SPRAINS 72
STOMACH UPSET 10,72
STREP THROAT 73
STROKES 62
STUTTERING 73
SUNBURNS 73
SWELLING 73

T

TEETHING 10
THRUSH 10
TICK BITES 74
TOOTH CARE 75

U

ULCERS 75
UMBILICAL INFECTIONS
10

V

VARICOSE VEINS 76

W

WARTS 76
WEIGHT LOSS 81
WHOOPING COUGH 76
WHOOPING COUGH
MEDICINE 89
WILD CHERRY COUGH
SYRUP 89
WOUNDS 76

Y

YEAST INFECTION 10,80

1st Printing 2001 2M 1st Edition
2nd Printing 2001 2M 1st Edition
3rd Printing 2001 3.5M 1st Edition
4th Printing 2001 5.5M 1st Edition
5th Printing 2002 12M Revised & Expanded 3rd Edition
6th Printing 2003 20M Slightly Revised
7th Printing 2004 25M Revised & Expanded 4th Edition
8th Printing 2005 30M Revised & Expanded 5th Edition
9th Printing 2008 10M Revised & Expanded 6th Edition

GIVE A GIFT THAT WILL BE APPRECIATED ALL YEAR!

HOME REMEDIES II FOR THE FARM, GARDEN, LAWN & HOUSE

For obtaining copies of this book, send check or money order to:
Abana Books Ltd 6523 Township Rd 346 Millersburg, OH 44654

Each copy is $10 postpaid to the same address.

	Qty	Total
$10 X _____	=	_____
OH addresses add 7% sales tax		_____
Total =		_____

Name _____

Address _____

City / State / Zip _____

❑ Please send me information on how I can retail this book at my place of business.

(Cut or Copy)————✄————————————————————————

HOME REMEDIES FROM AMISH COUNTRY

(HR)

For obtaining copies of this book, send check or money order to:
Abana Books Ltd 6523 Township Rd 346 Millersburg, OH 44654

Each copy is $10 postpaid to the same address.

	Qty	Total
$10 X _____	=	_____
OH addresses add 7% sales tax		_____
Total =		_____

Name _____

Address _____

City / State / Zip _____

❑ Please send me information on how I can retail this book at my place of business.

GIVE A GIFT THAT WILL BE APPRECIATED ALL YEAR!

HOME REMEDIES FROM AMISH COUNTRY

(HR)

For obtaining copies of this book, send check or money order to:
Abana Books Ltd 6523 Township Rd 346 Millersburg, OH 44654

Each copy is $10 postpaid to the same address.

Qty   Total

$10 X _____ = _____

OH addresses add 7% sales tax _____

Total = _____

Name _____

Address _____

City / State / Zip _____

❏ Please send me information on how I can retail this book at my place of business.

(Cut or Copy)————✂————————————————

HOME REMEDIES II FOR THE FARM, GARDEN, LAWN & HOUSE

For obtaining copies of this book, send check or money order to:
Abana Books Ltd 6523 Township Rd 346 Millersburg, OH 44654

Each copy is $10 postpaid to the same address.

Qty   Total

$10 X _____ = _____

OH addresses add 7% sales tax _____

Total = _____

Name _____

Address _____

City / State / Zip _____

❏ Please send me information on how I can retail this book at my place of business.